English Bulldog Dress-up

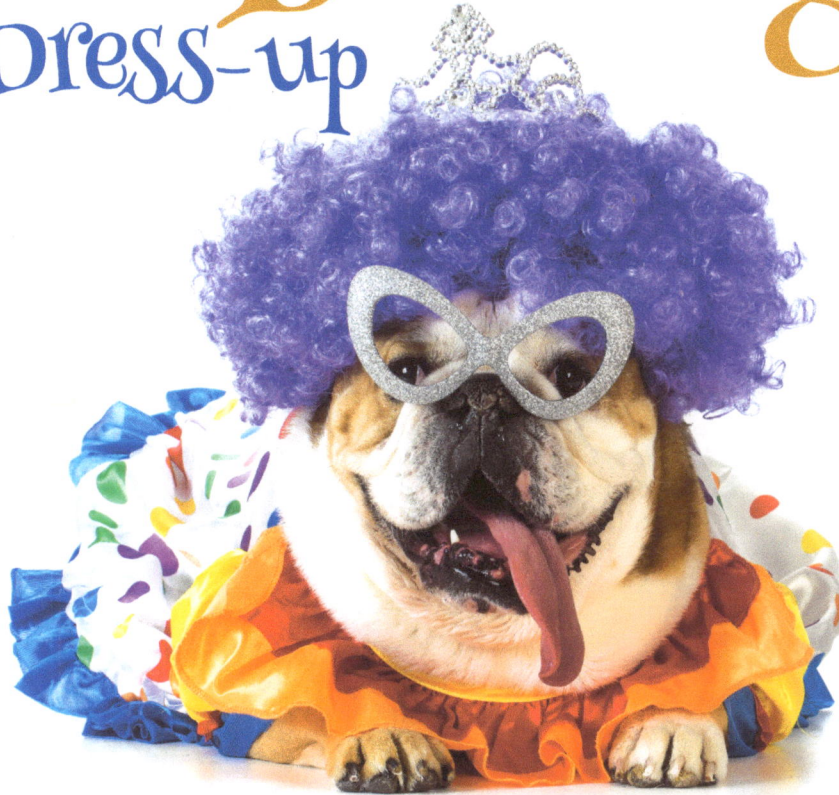

A No Text Picture Book

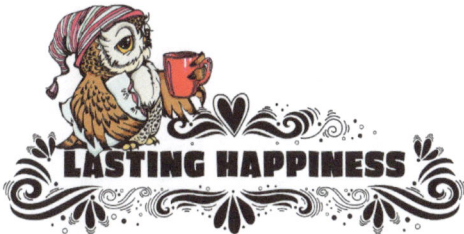

LASTING HAPPINESS

ISBN: 978-1-990181-23-8

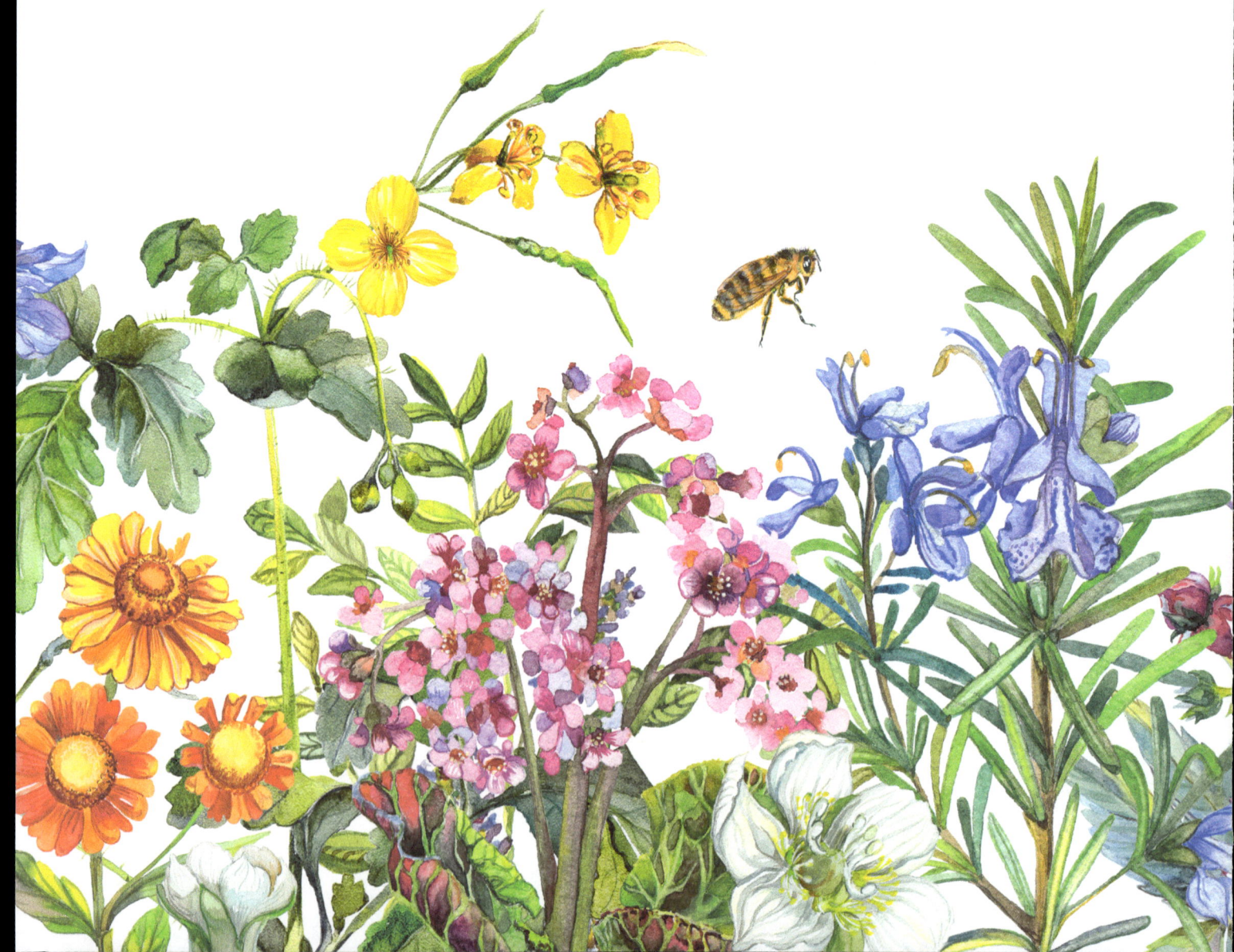

To:

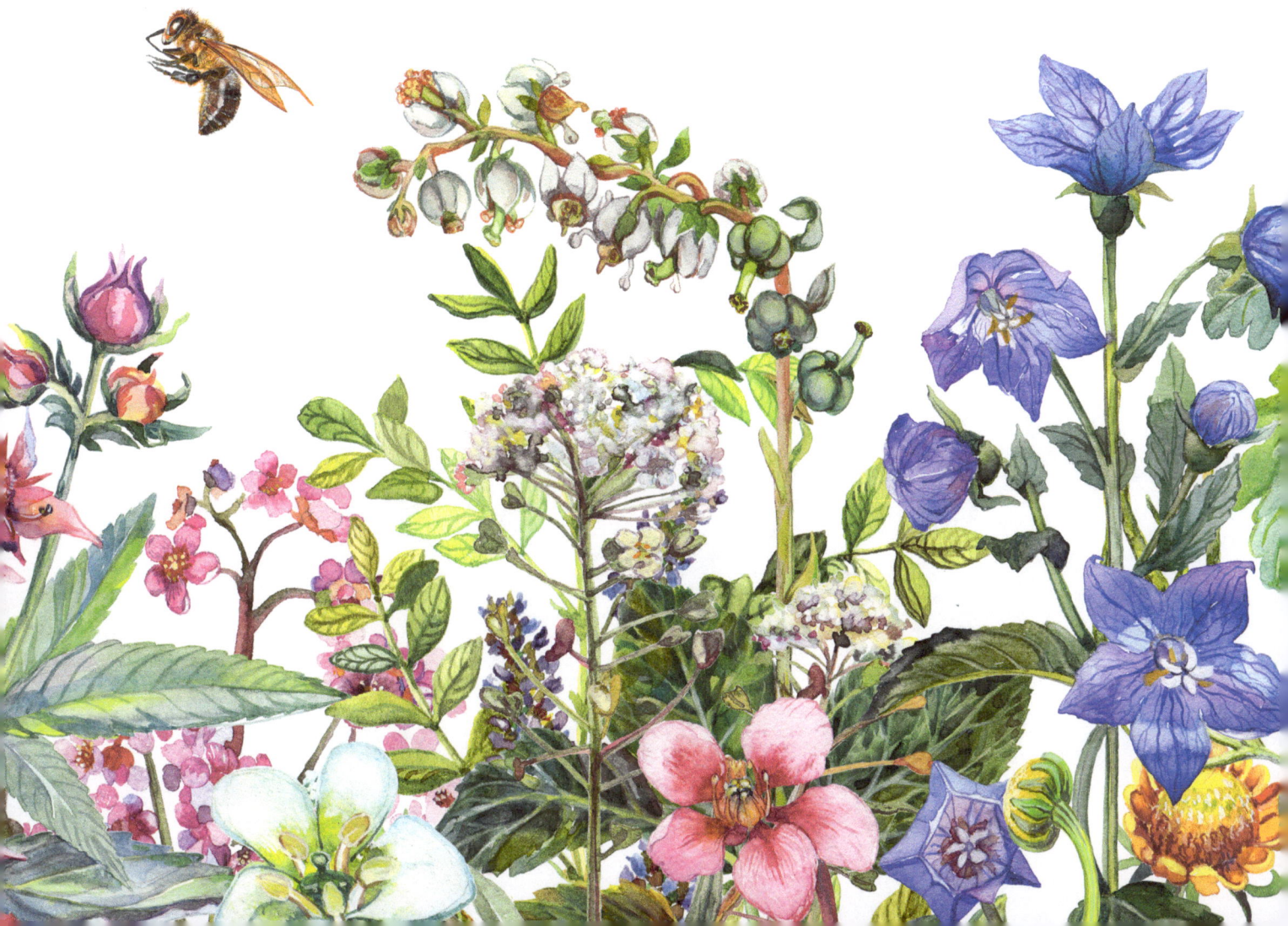

FROM:

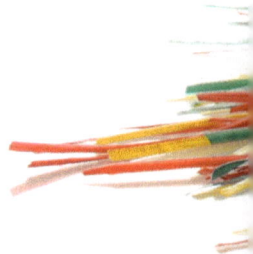

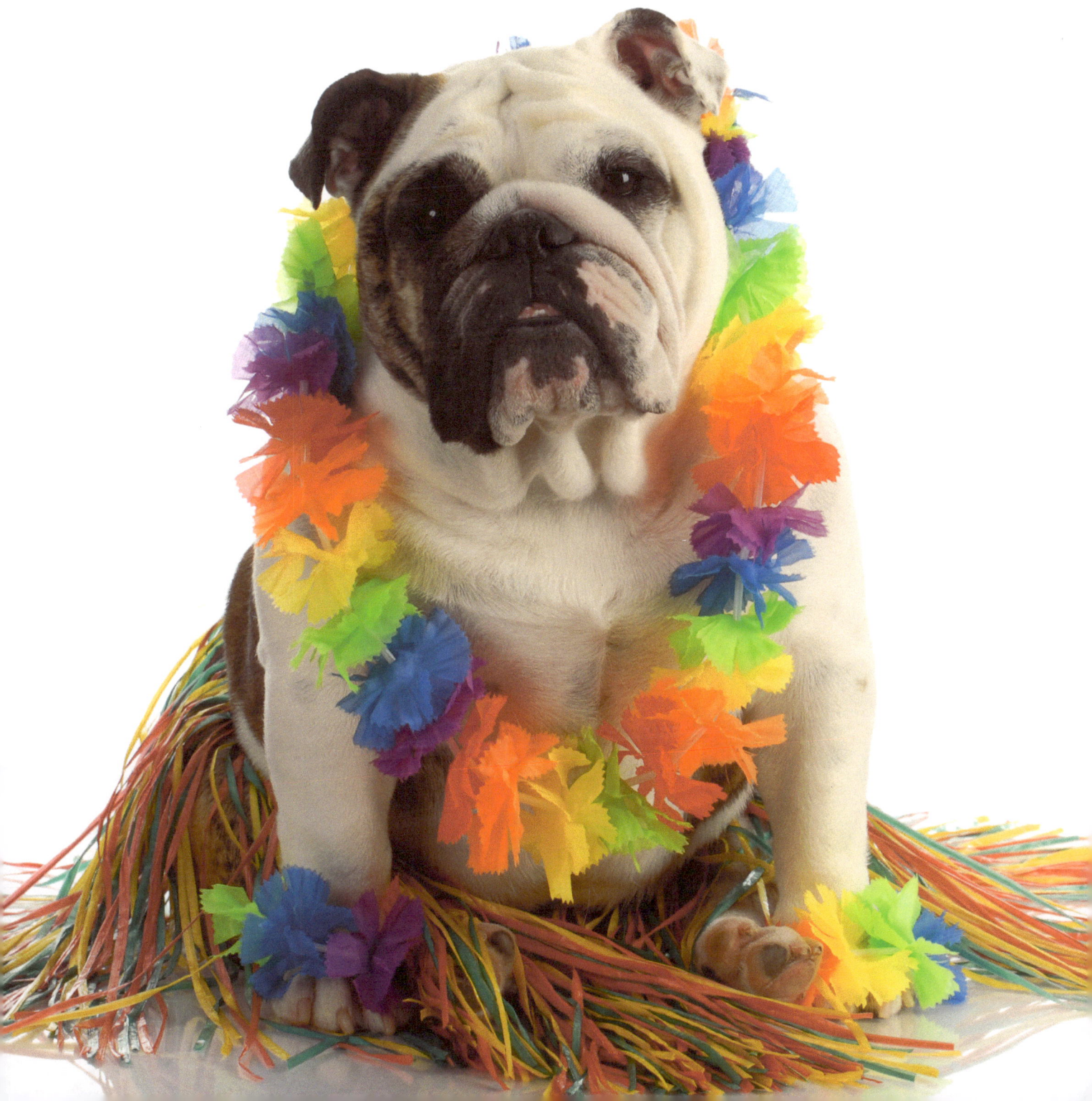

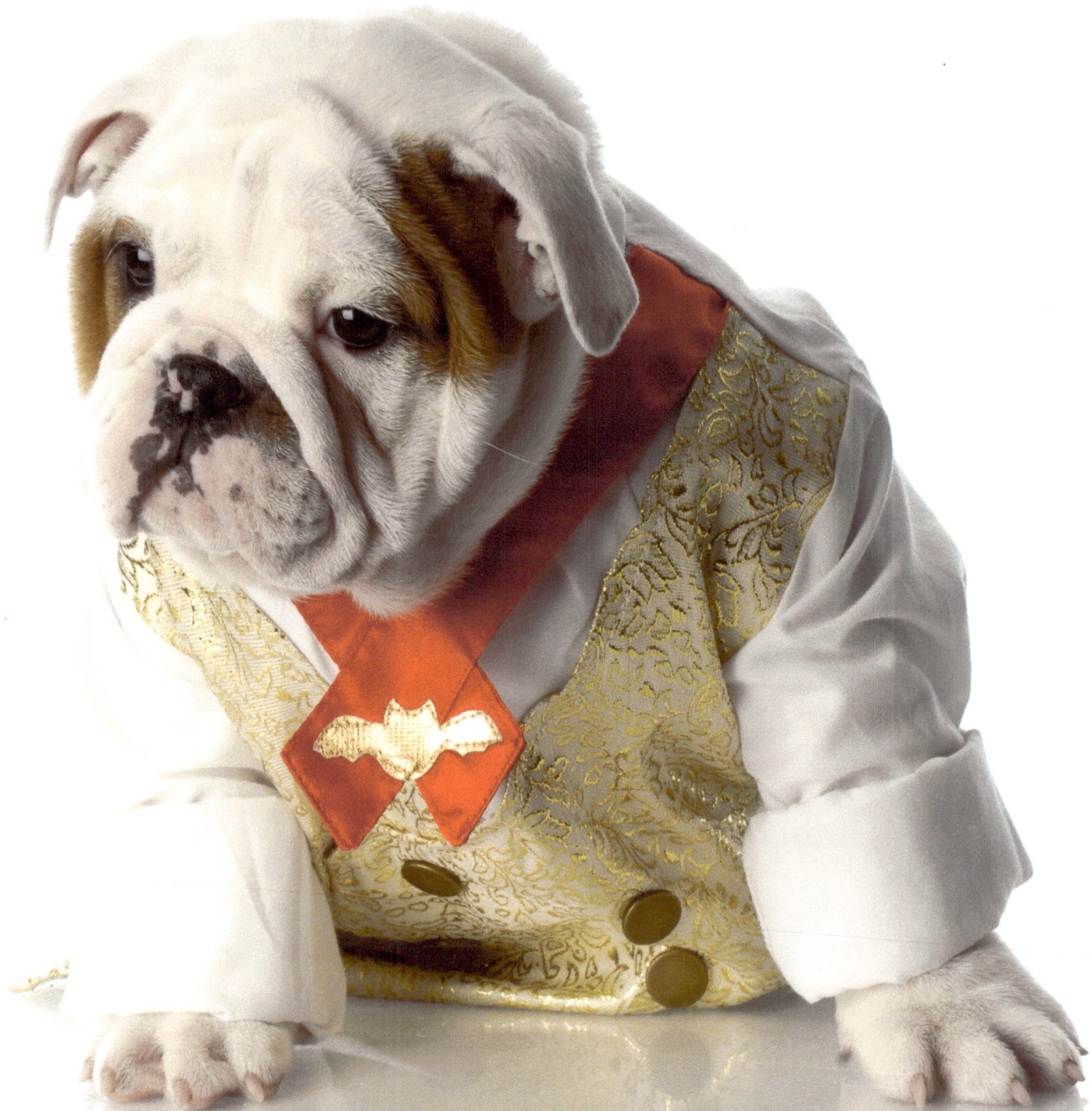

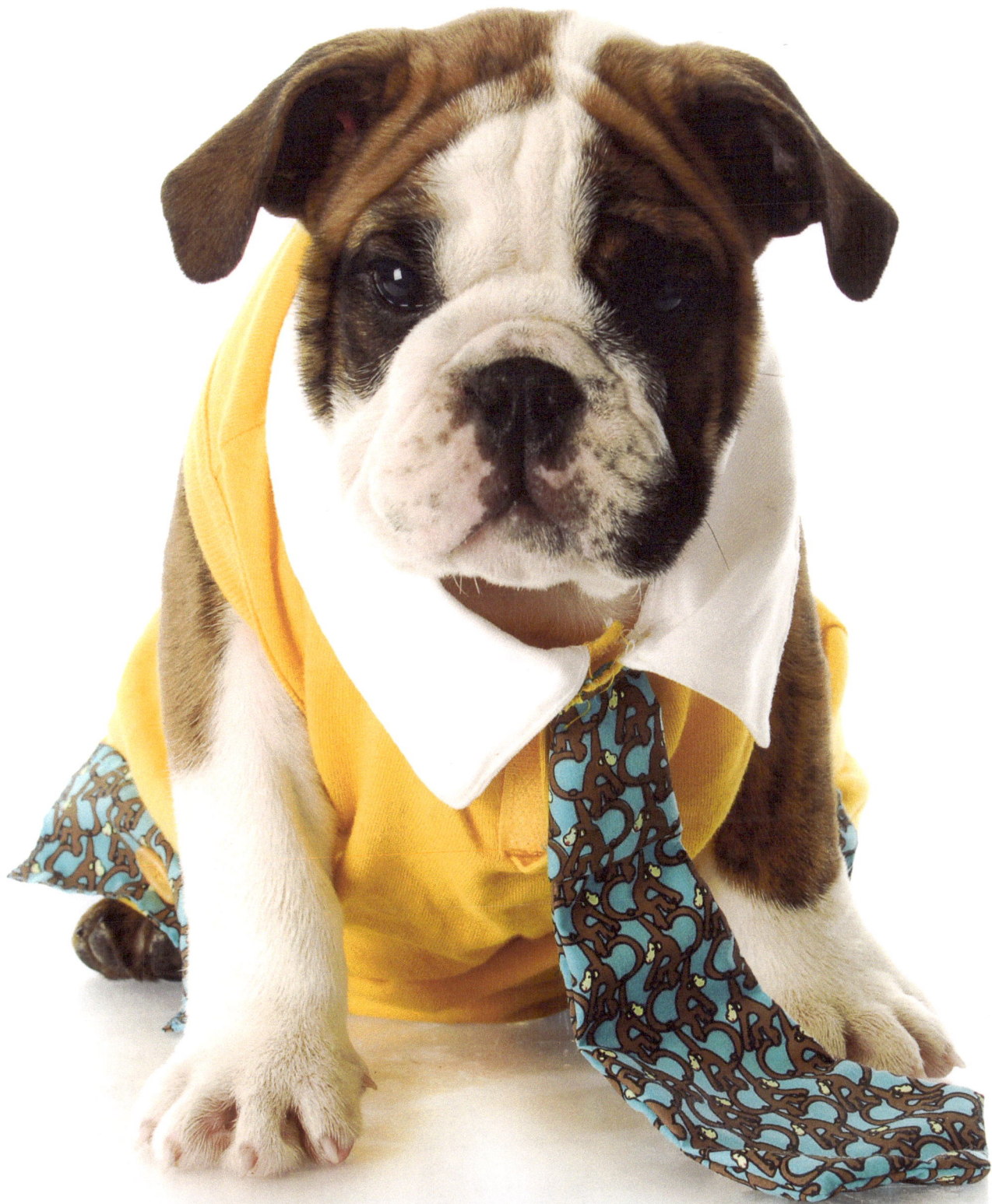

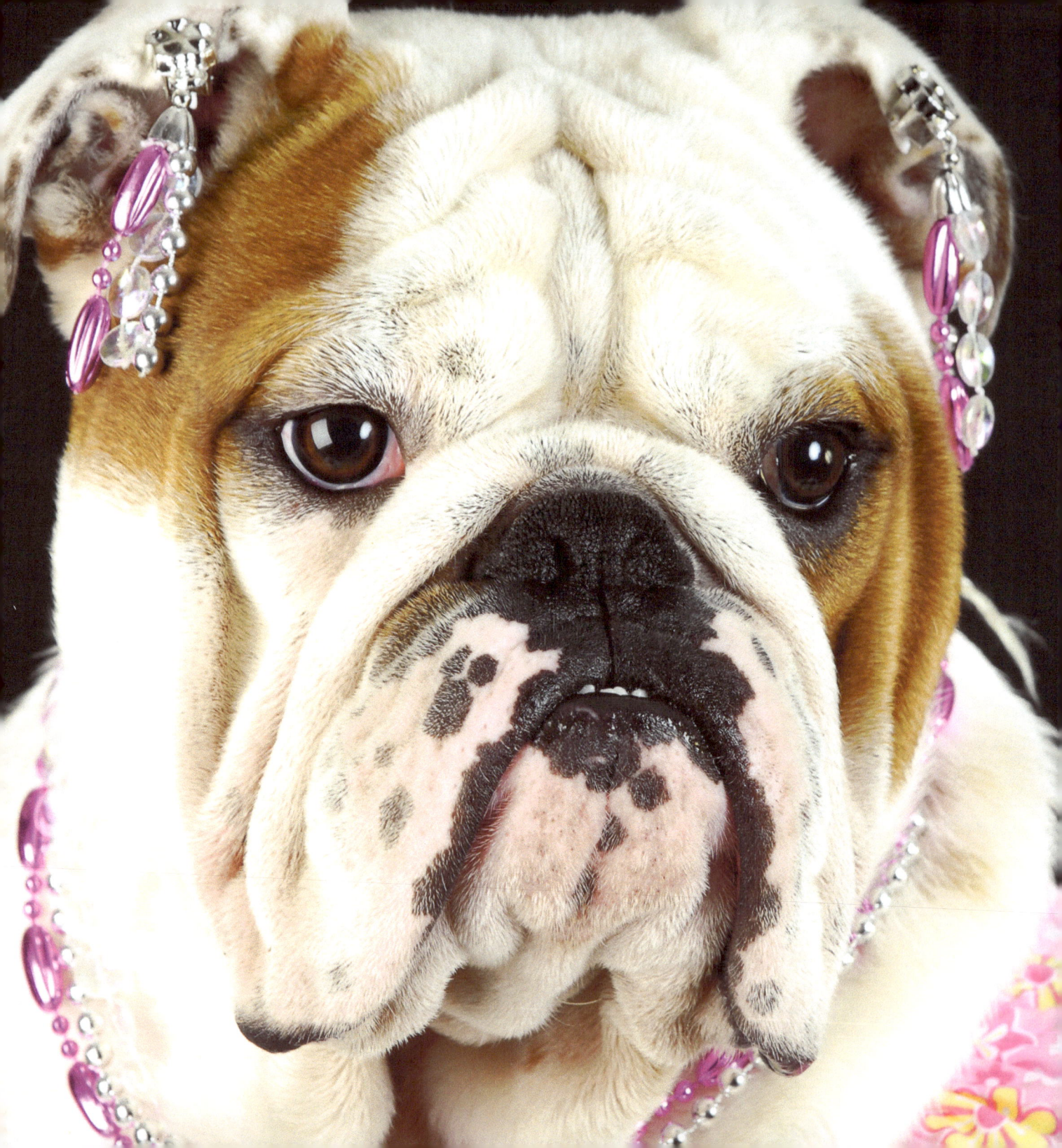

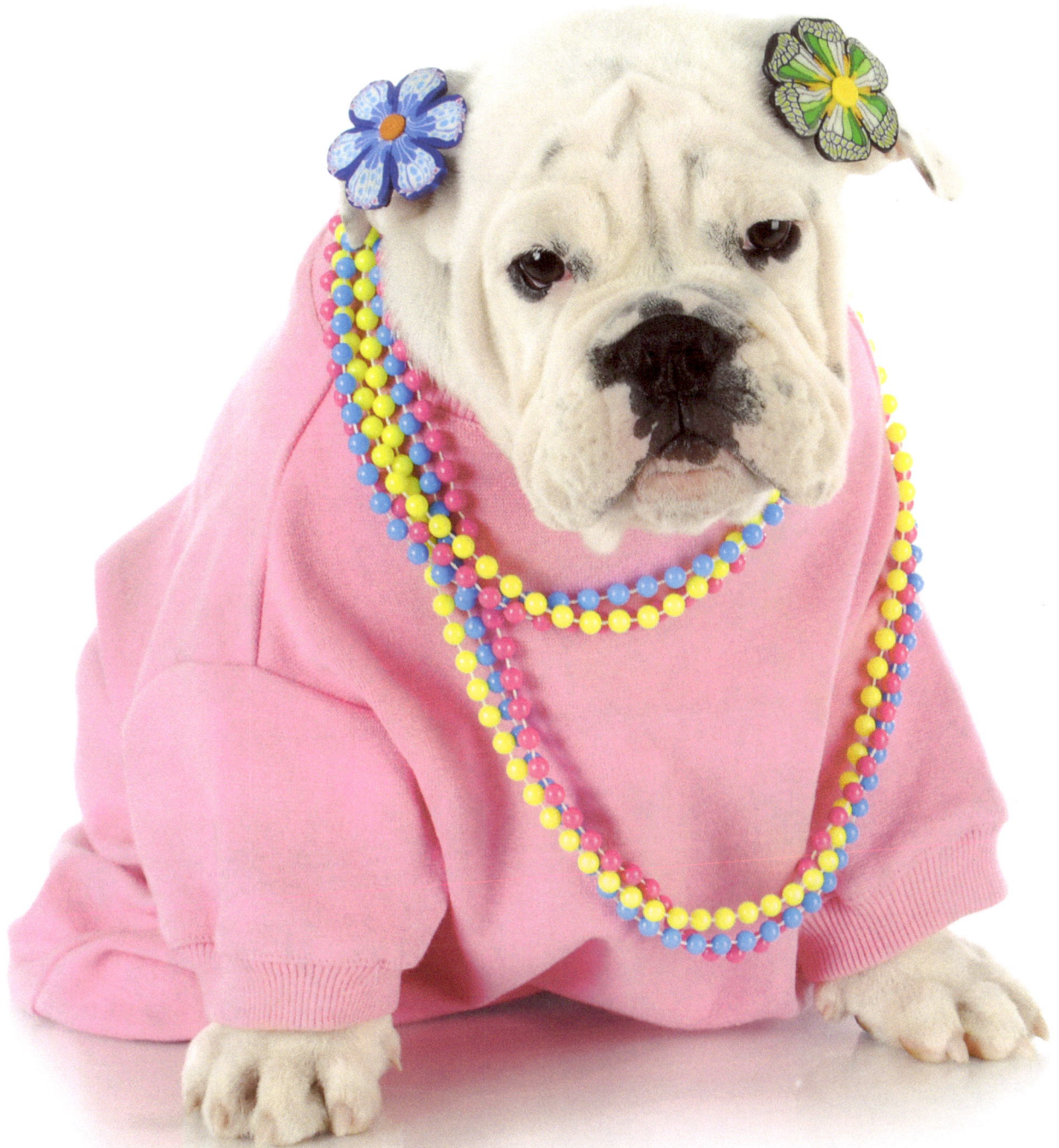

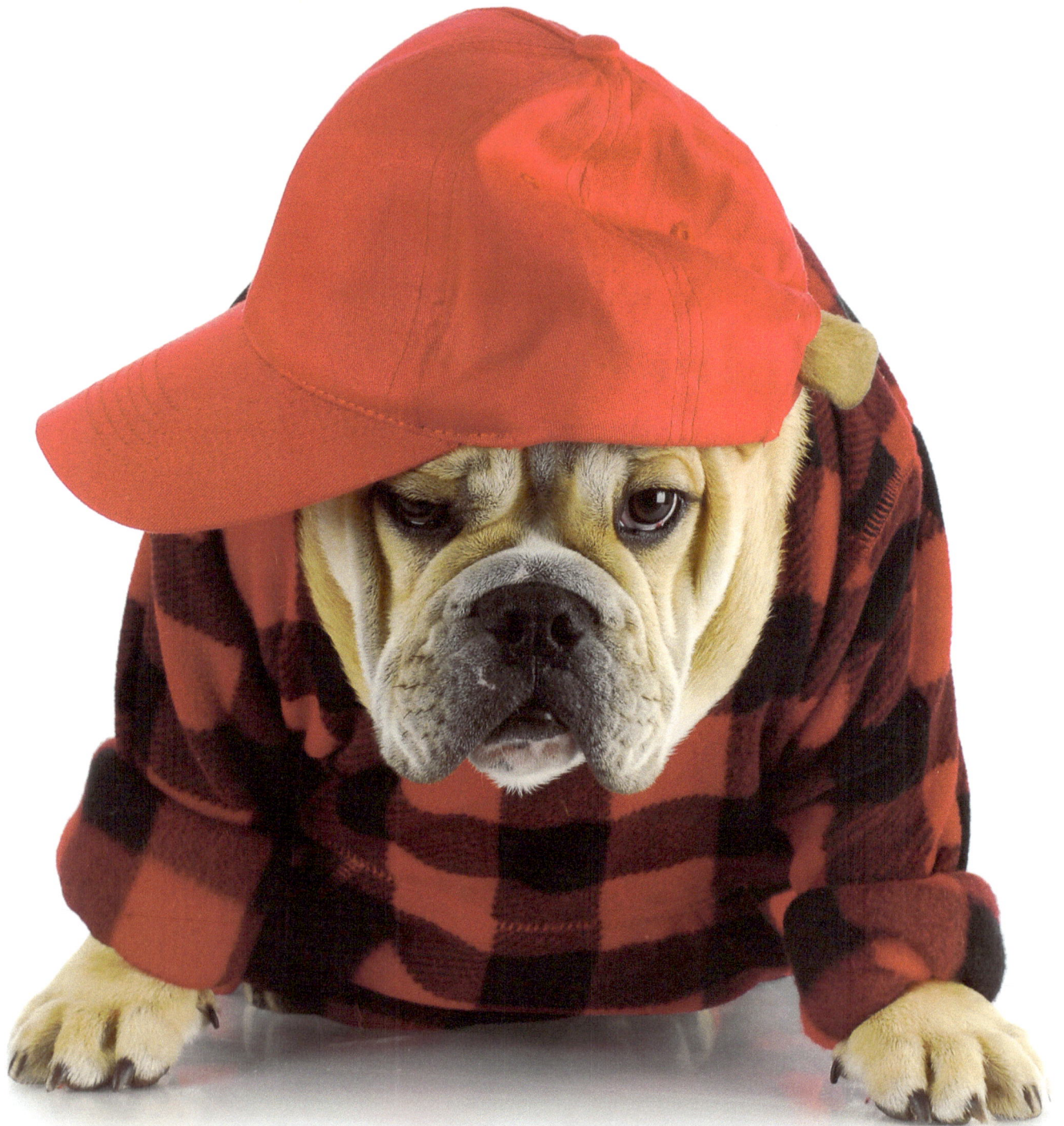

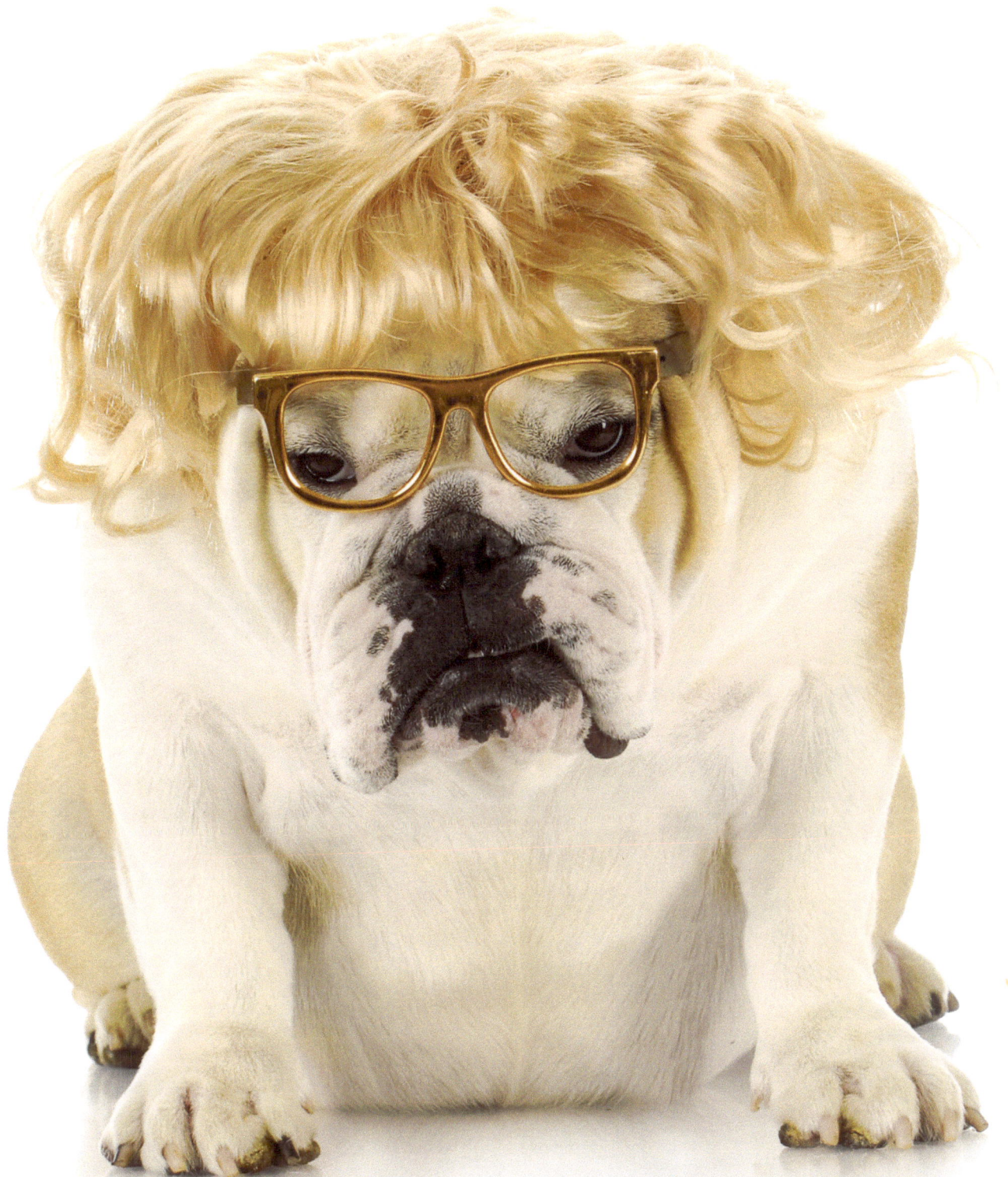

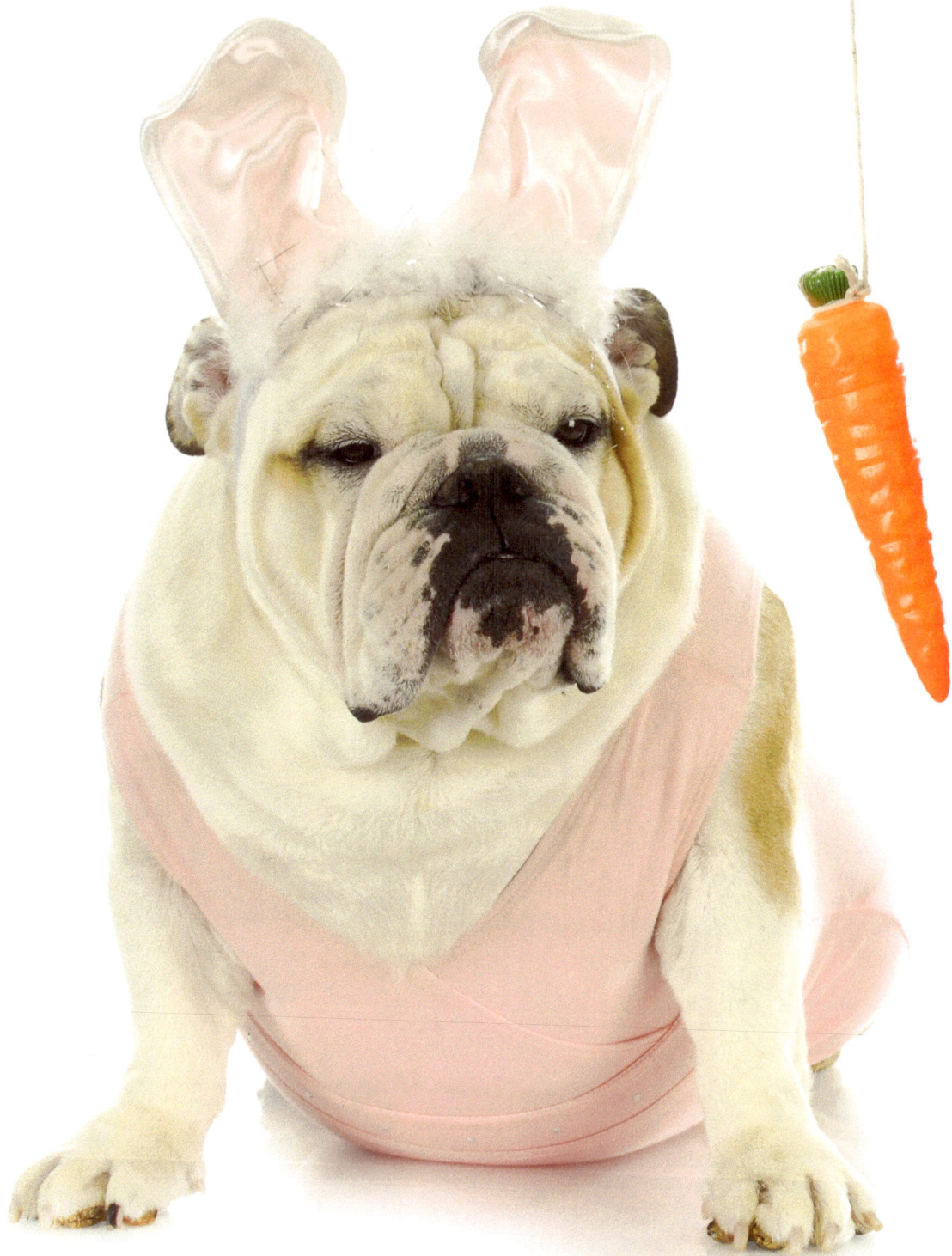

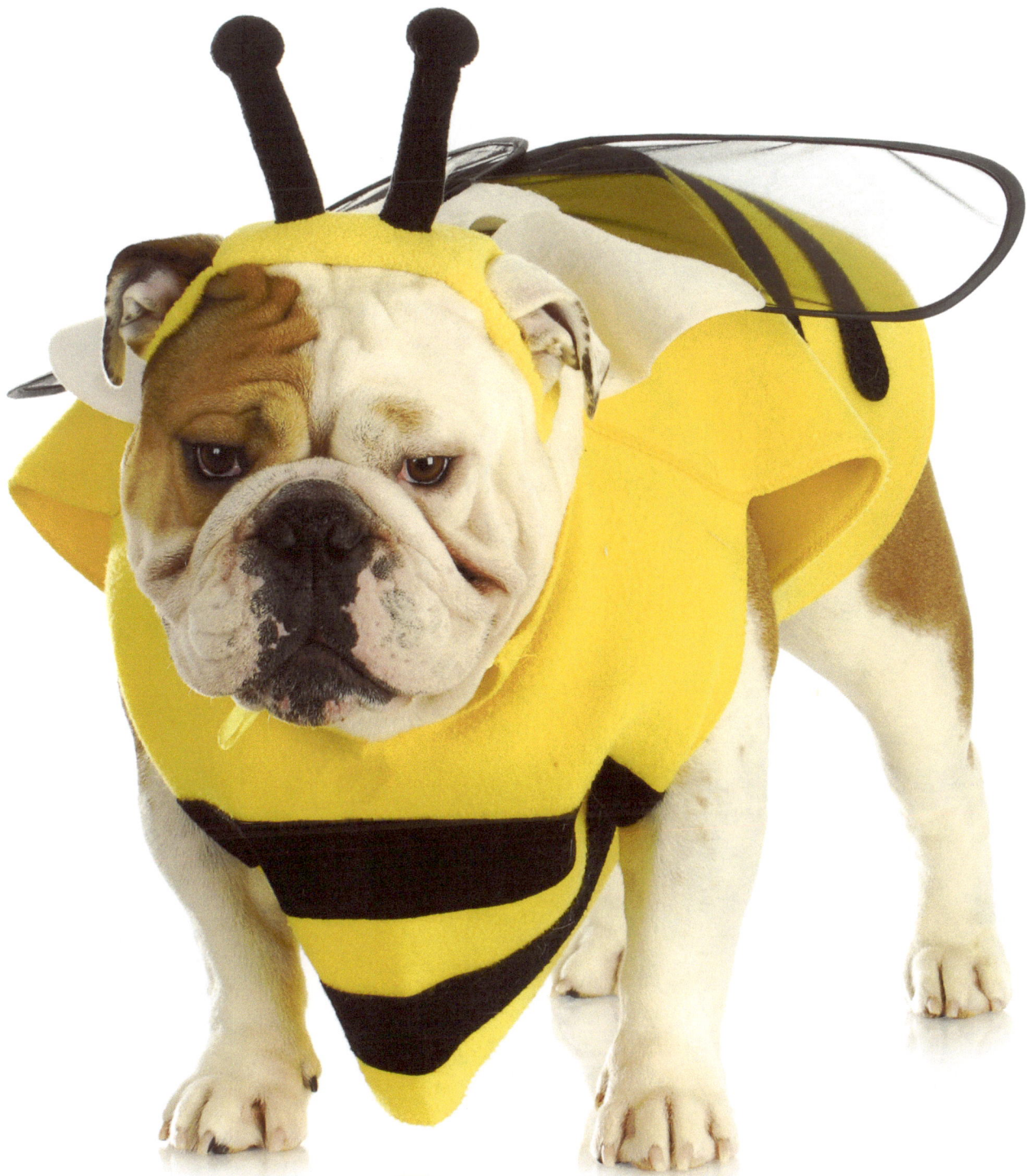

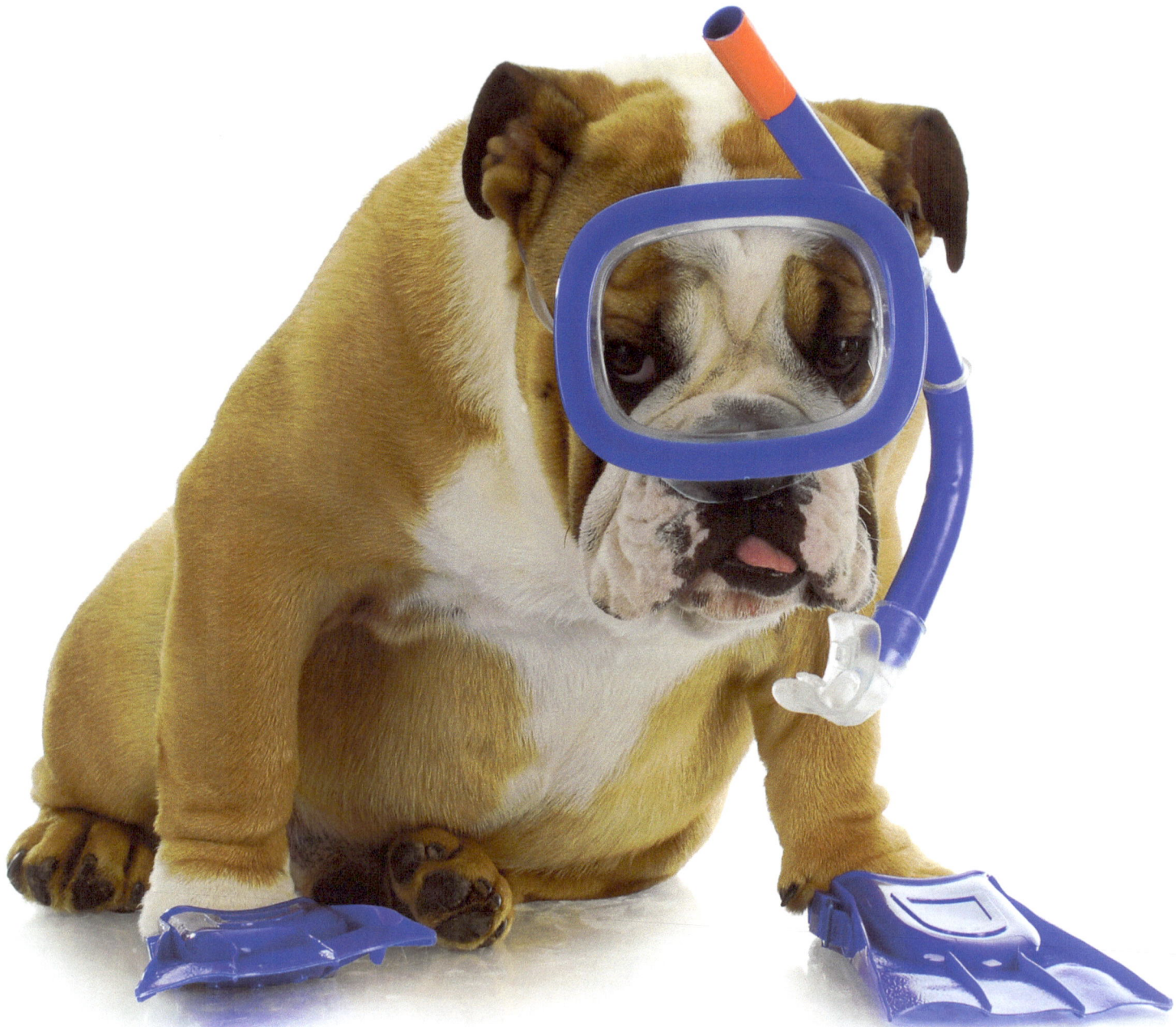

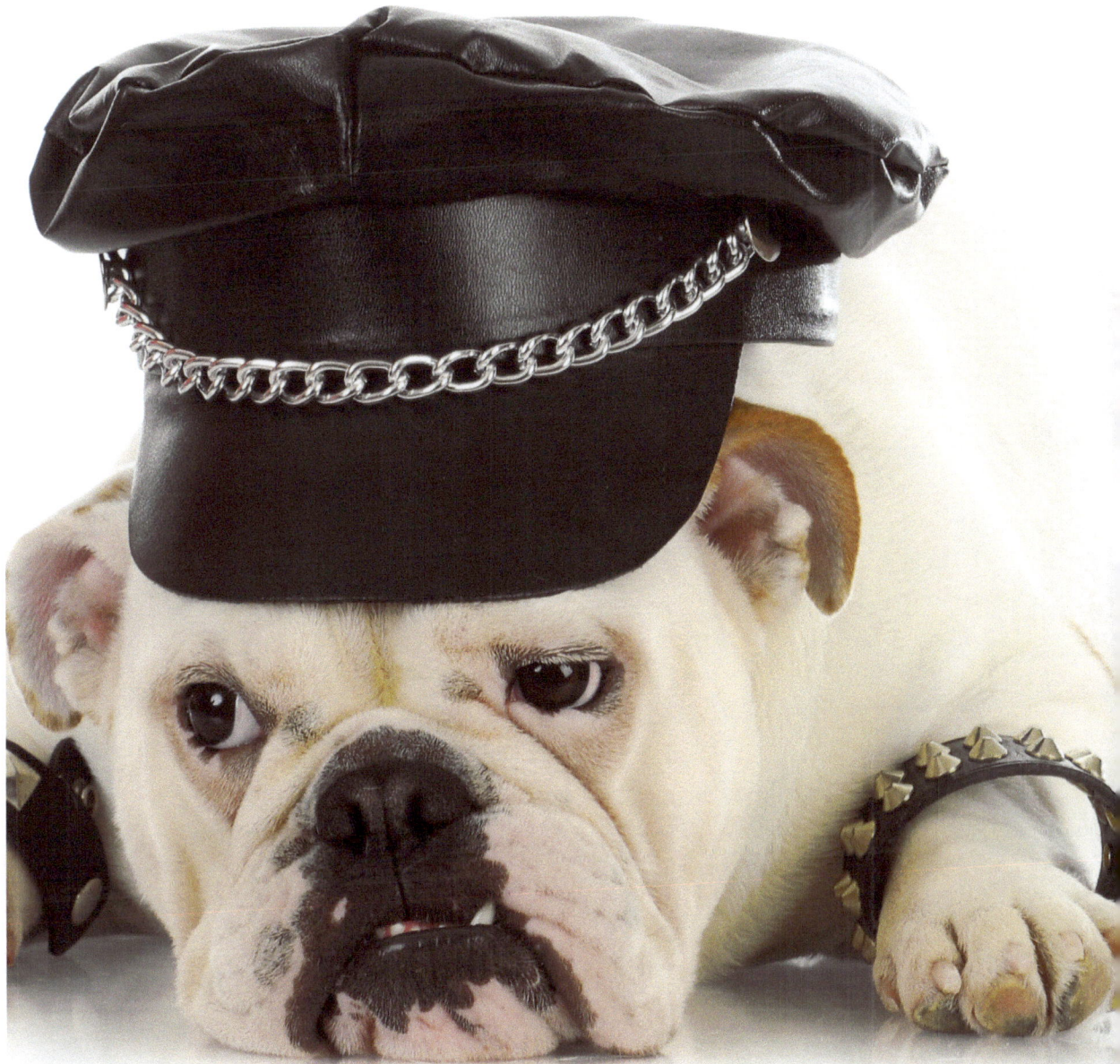

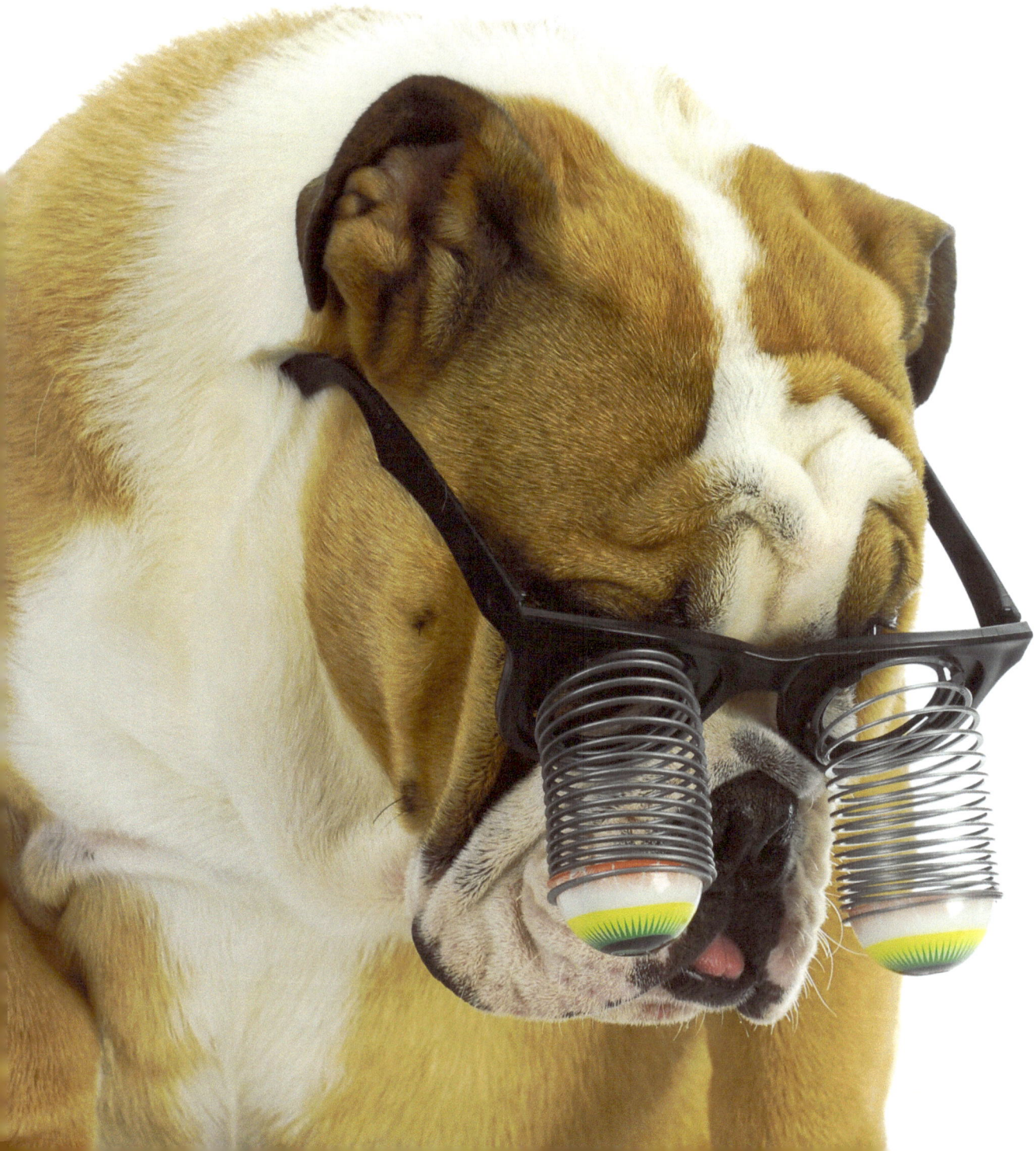

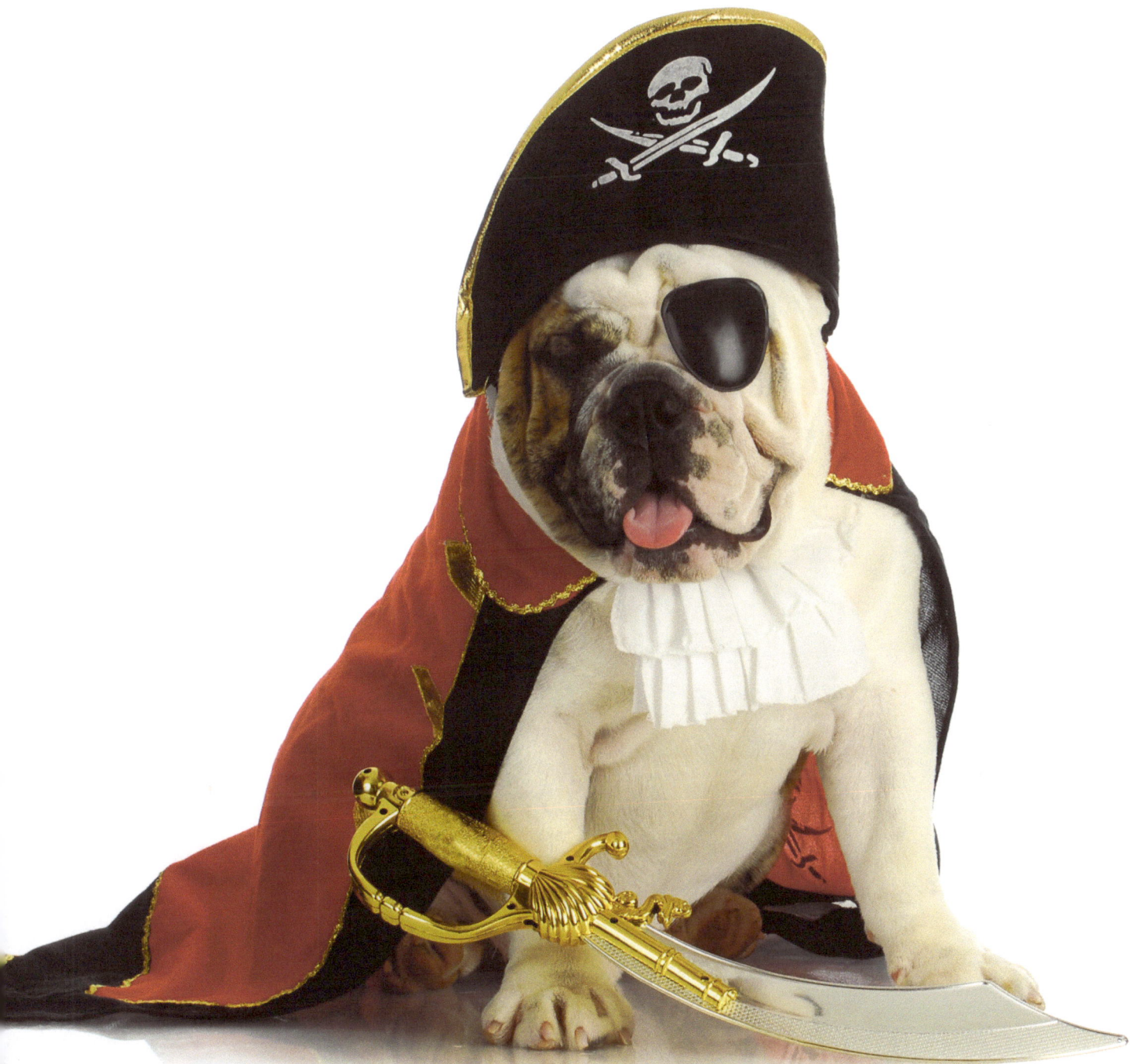

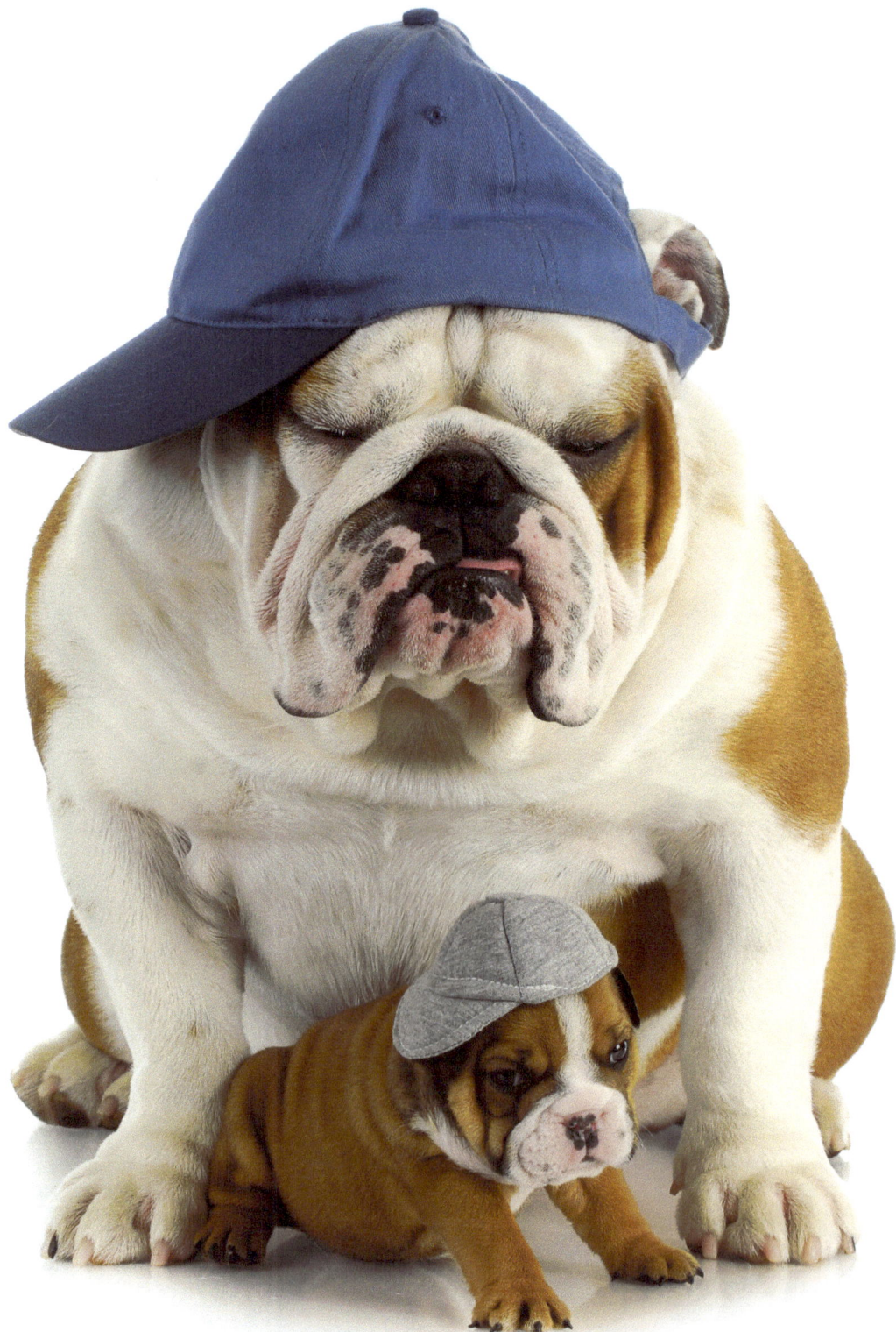

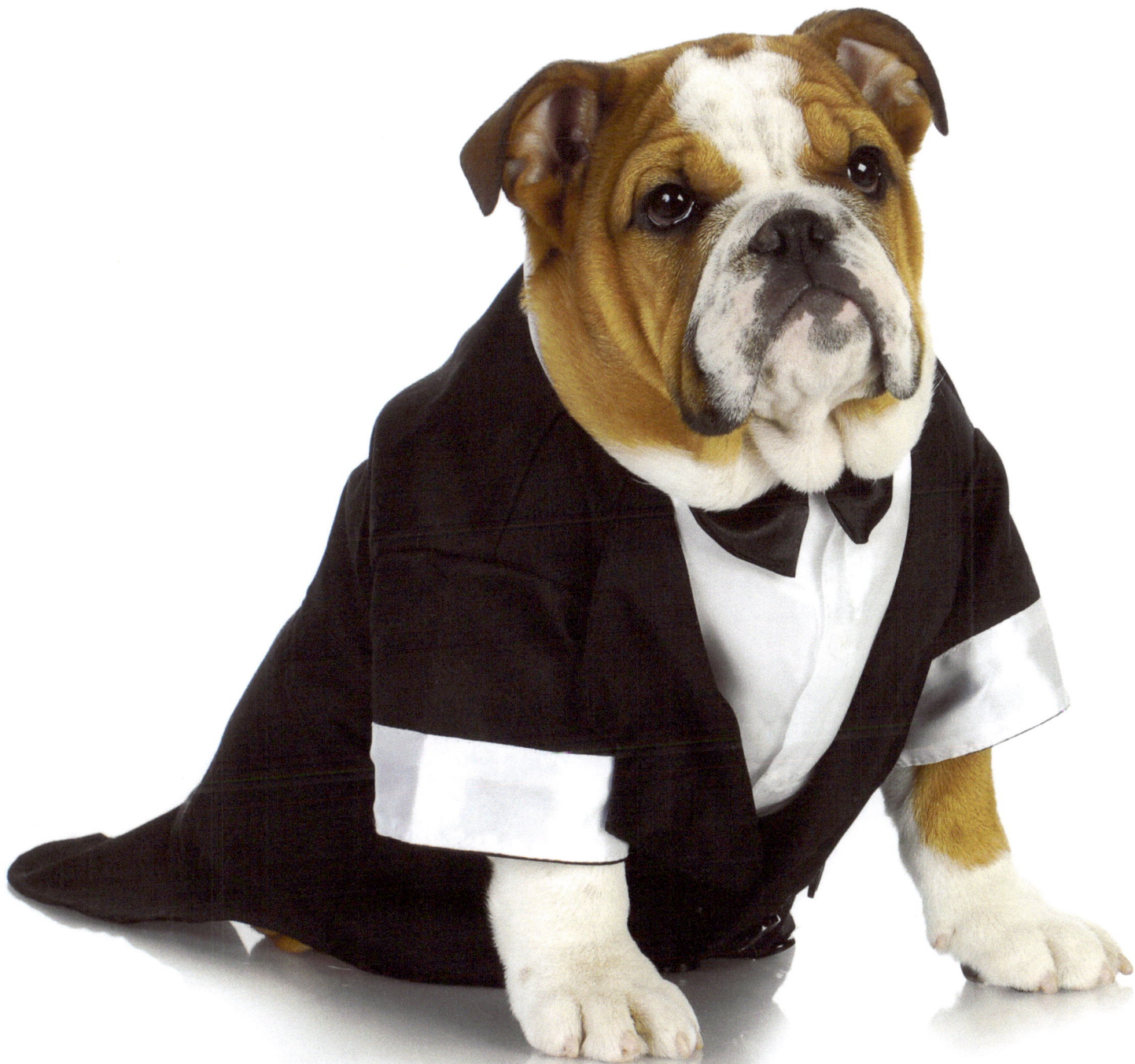

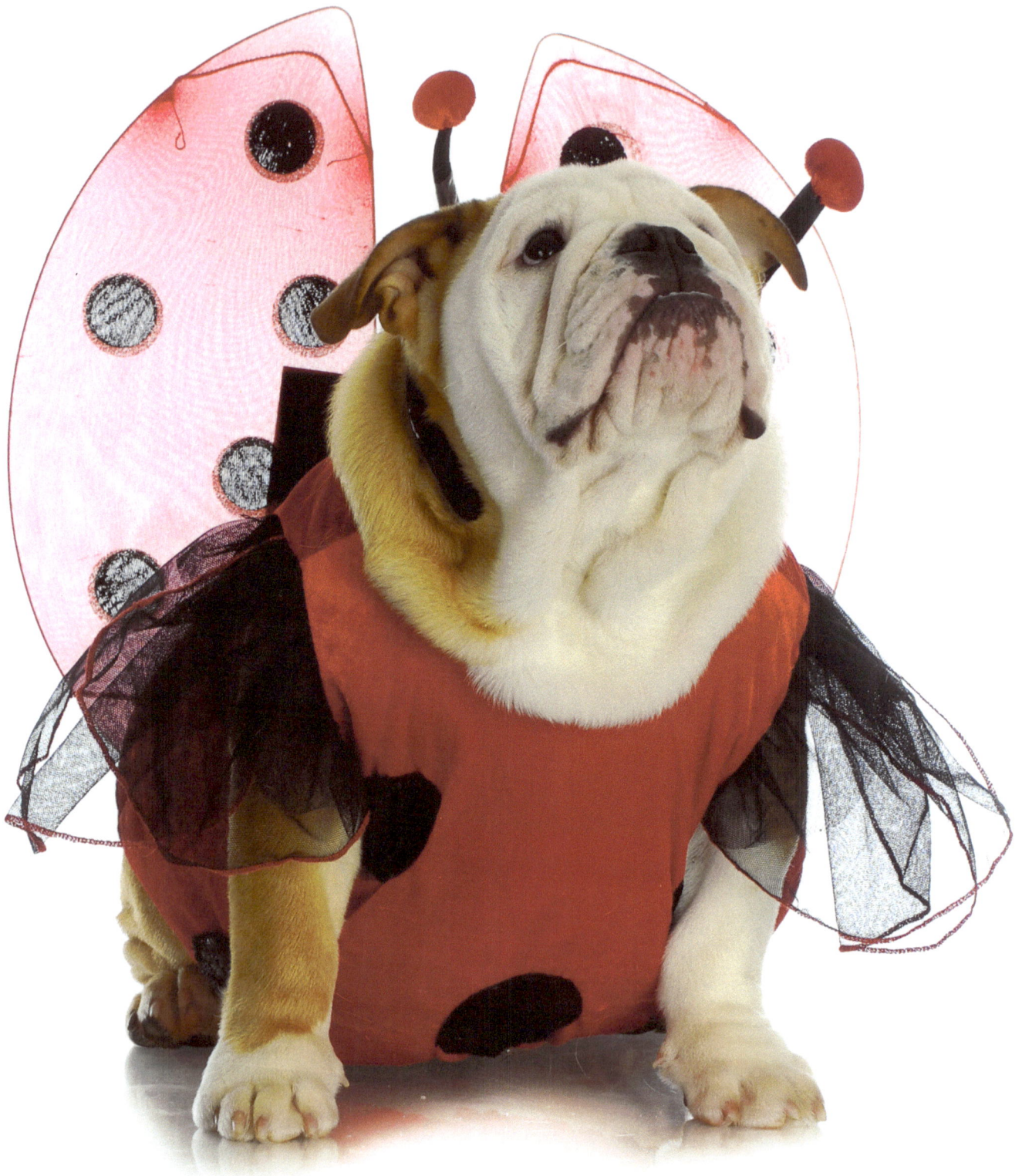

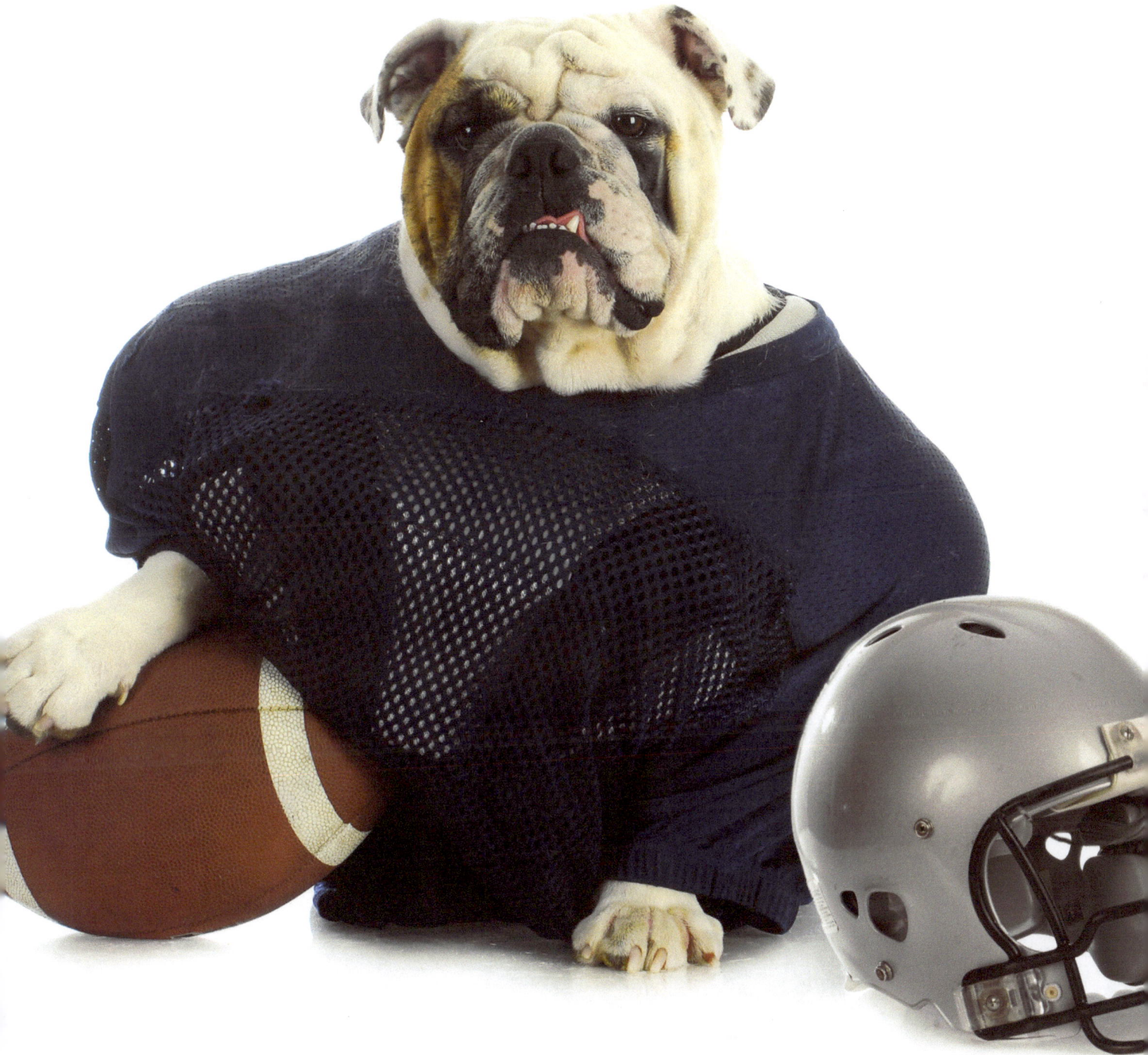

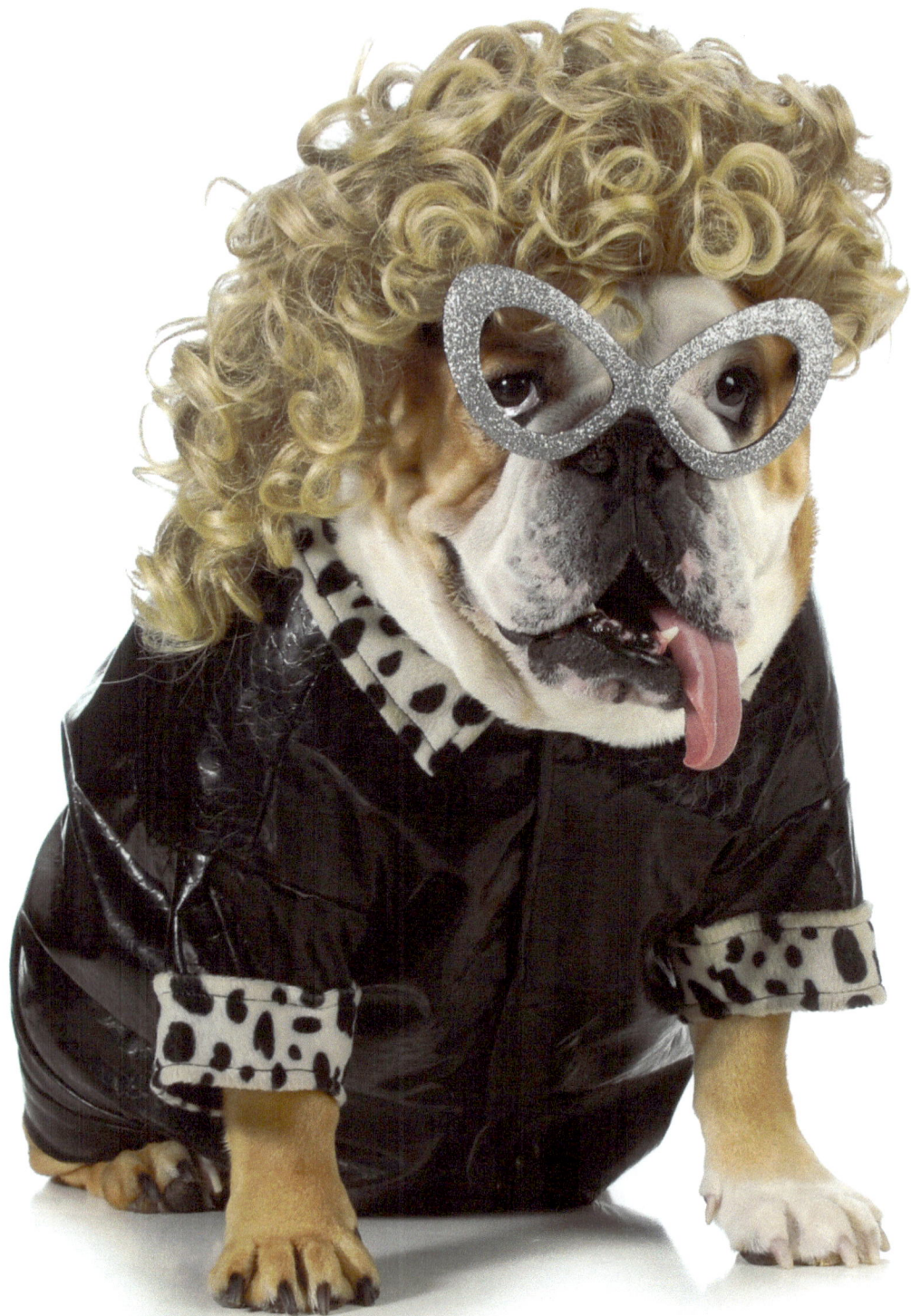

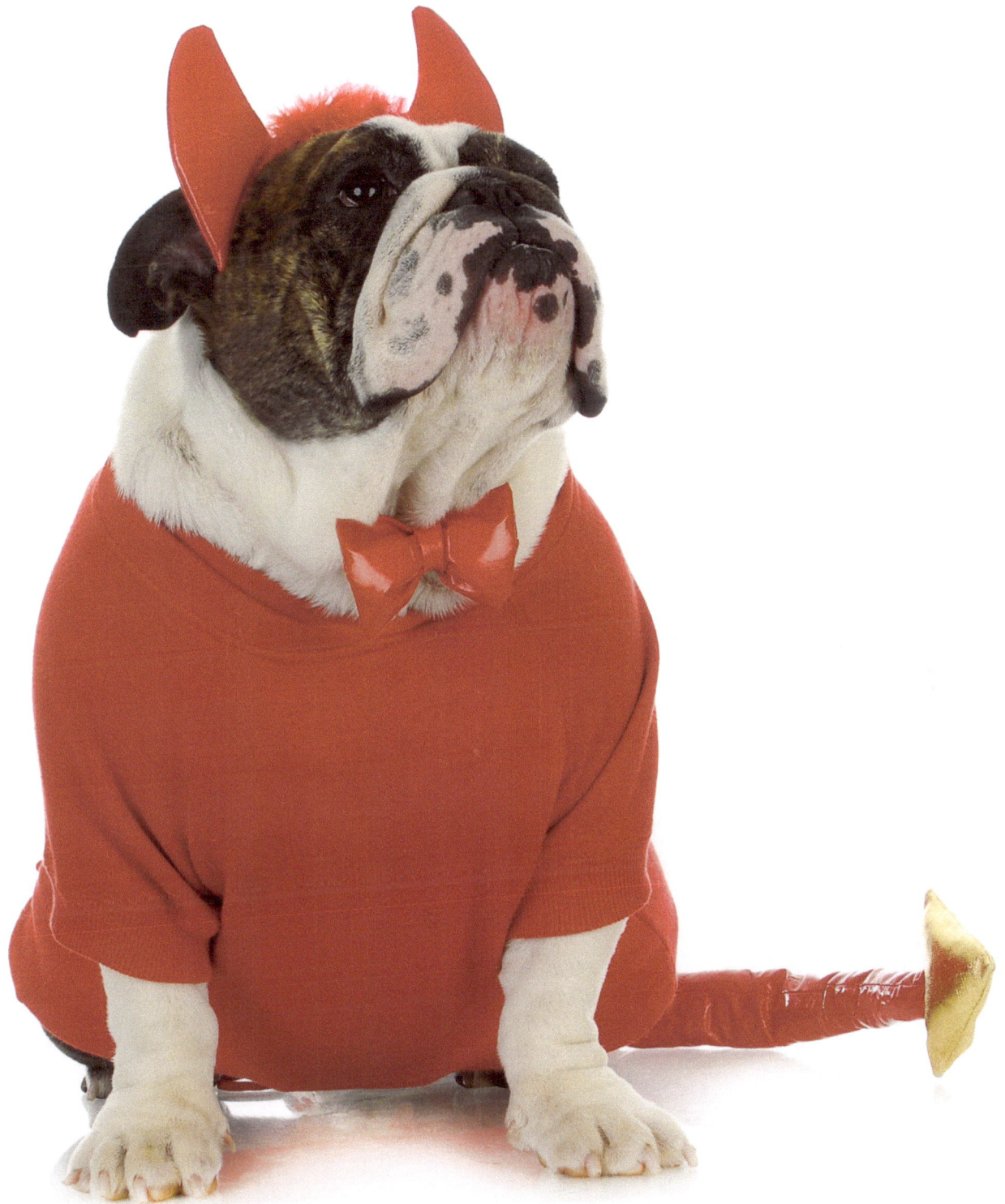

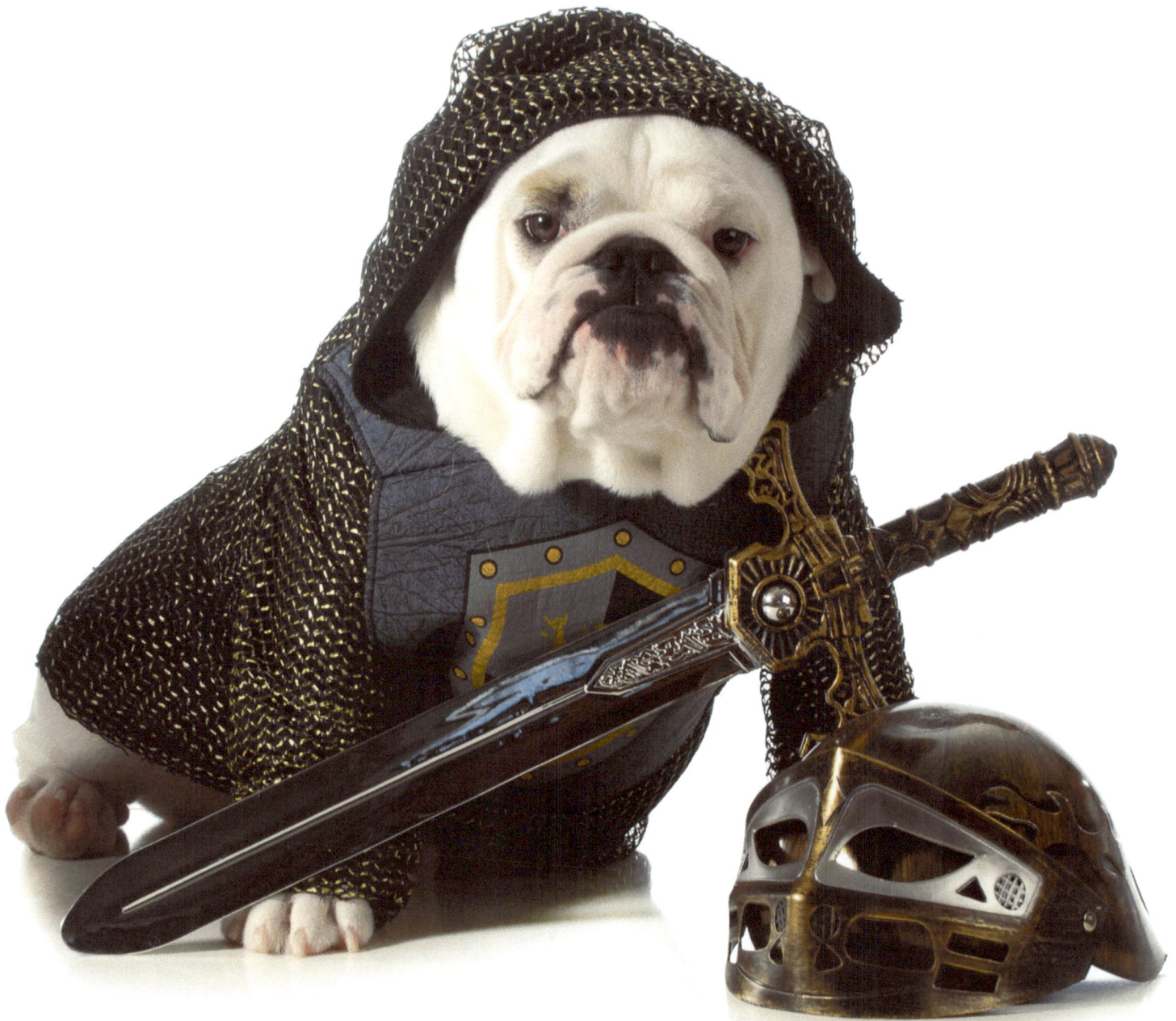

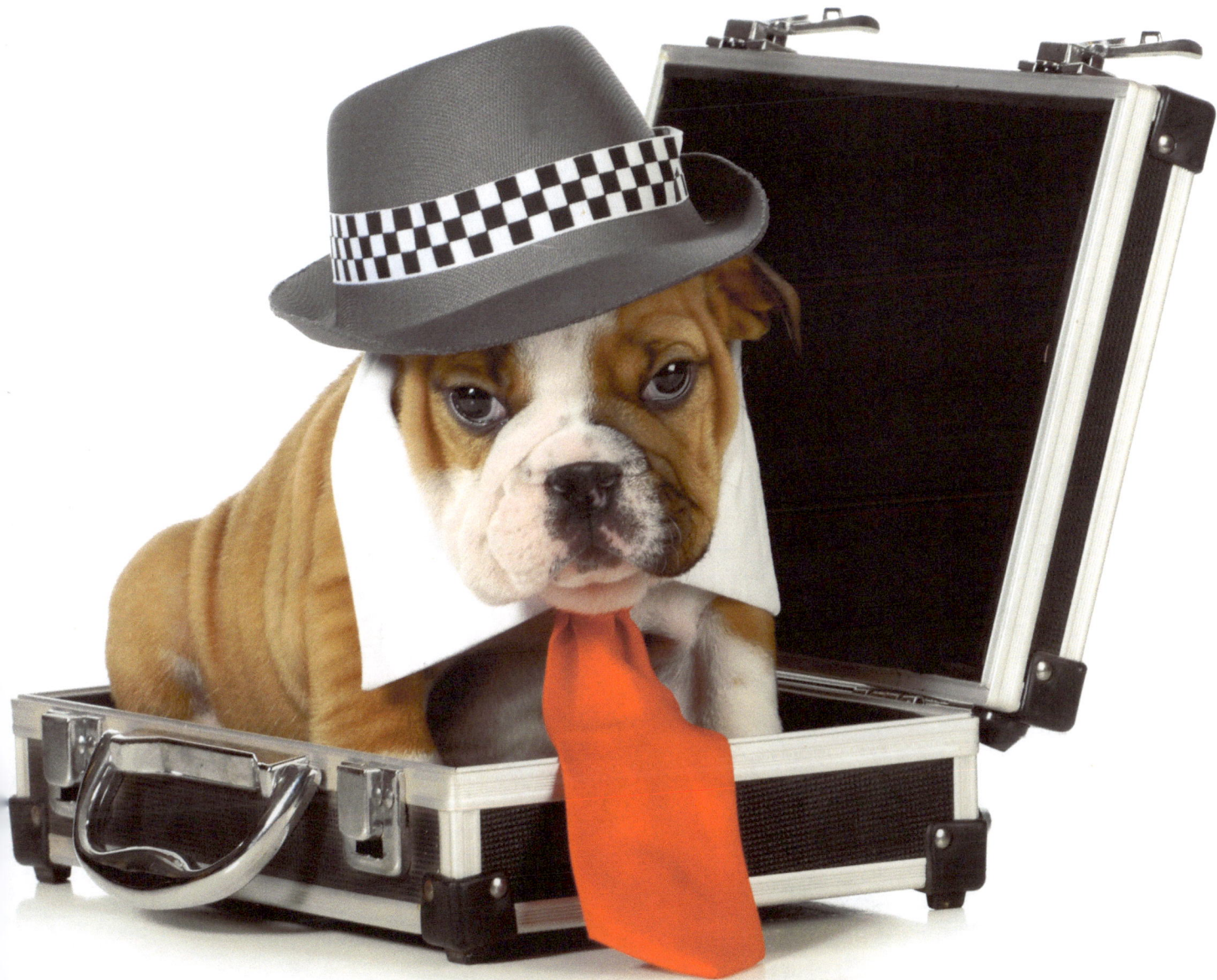

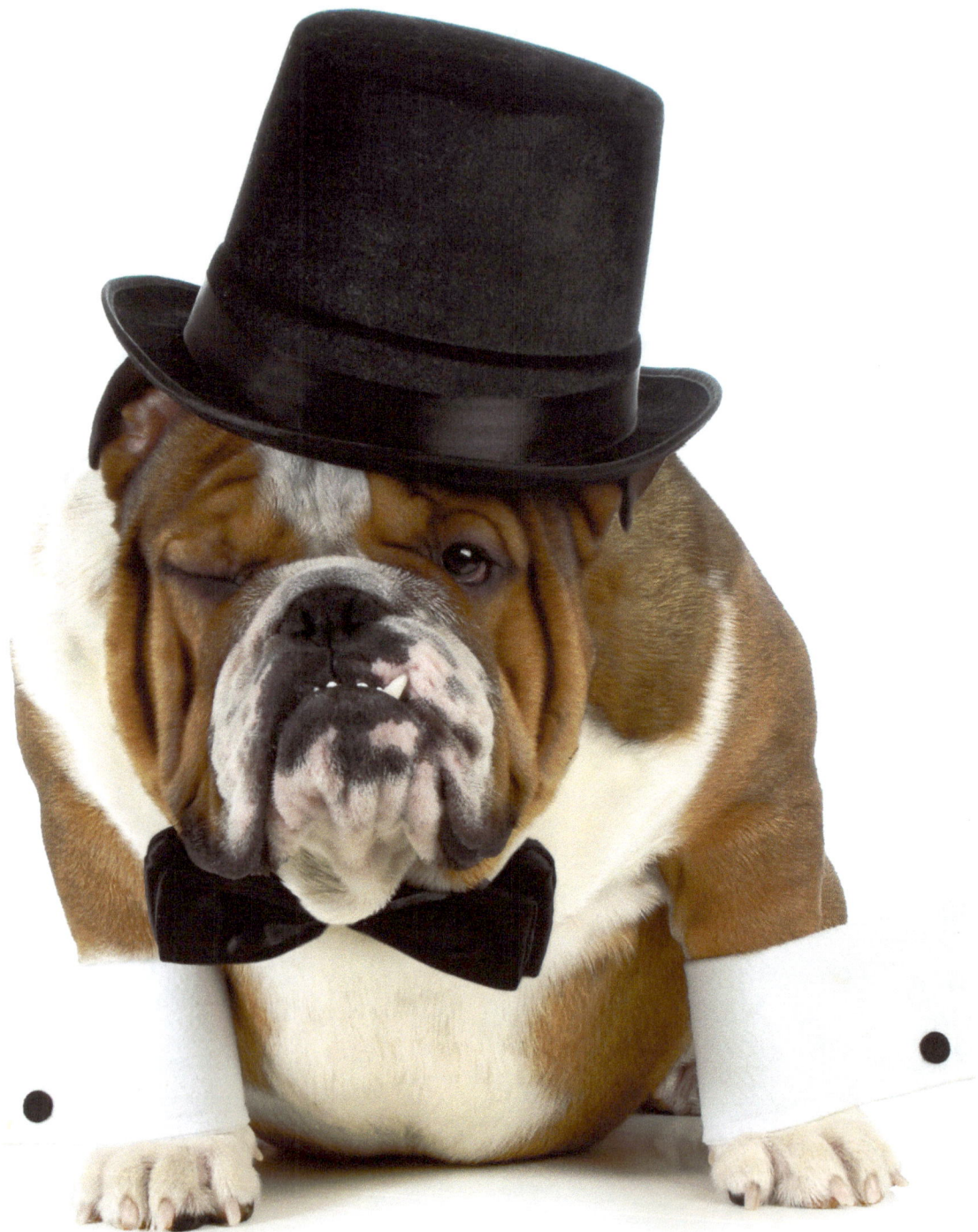

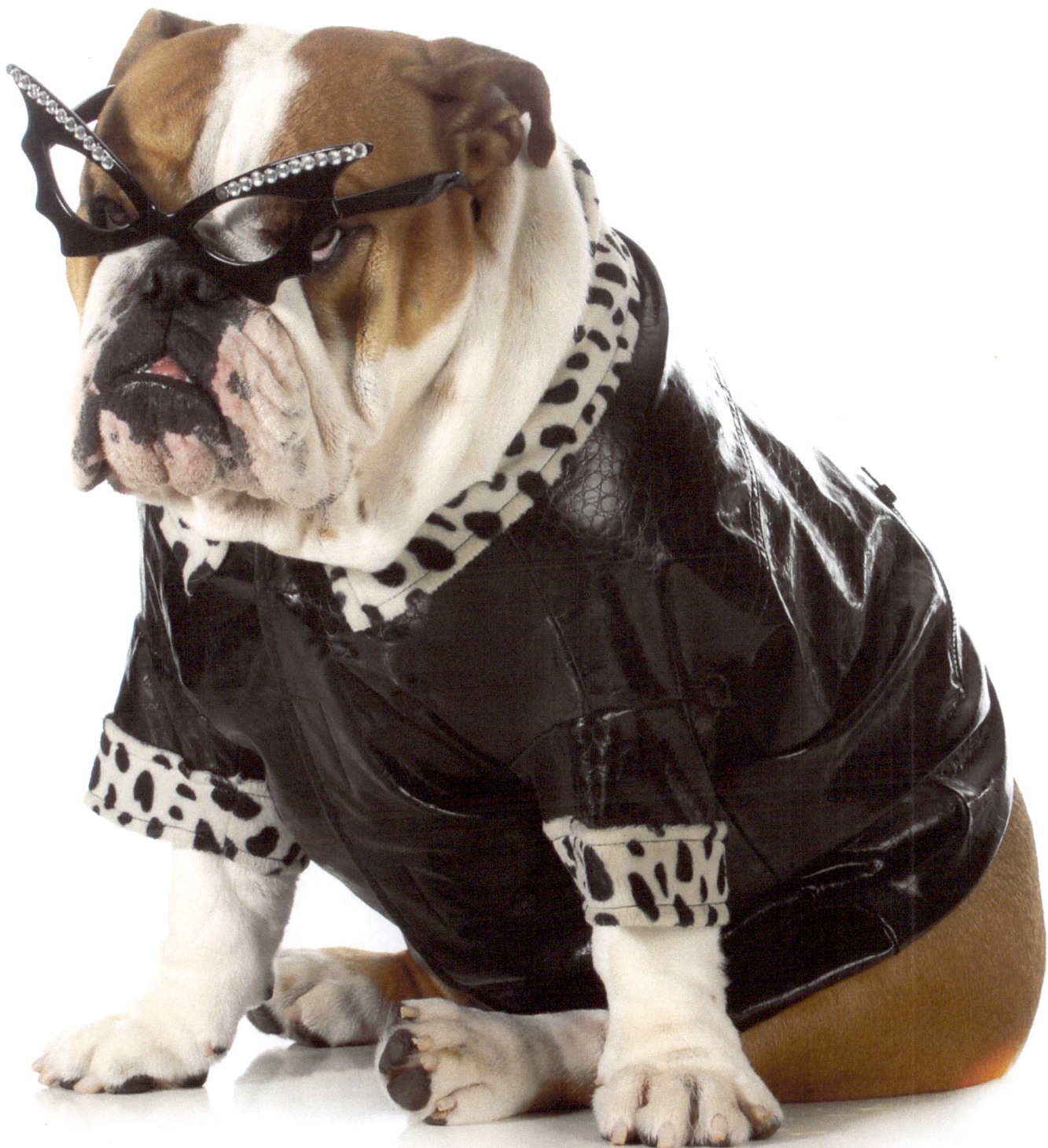

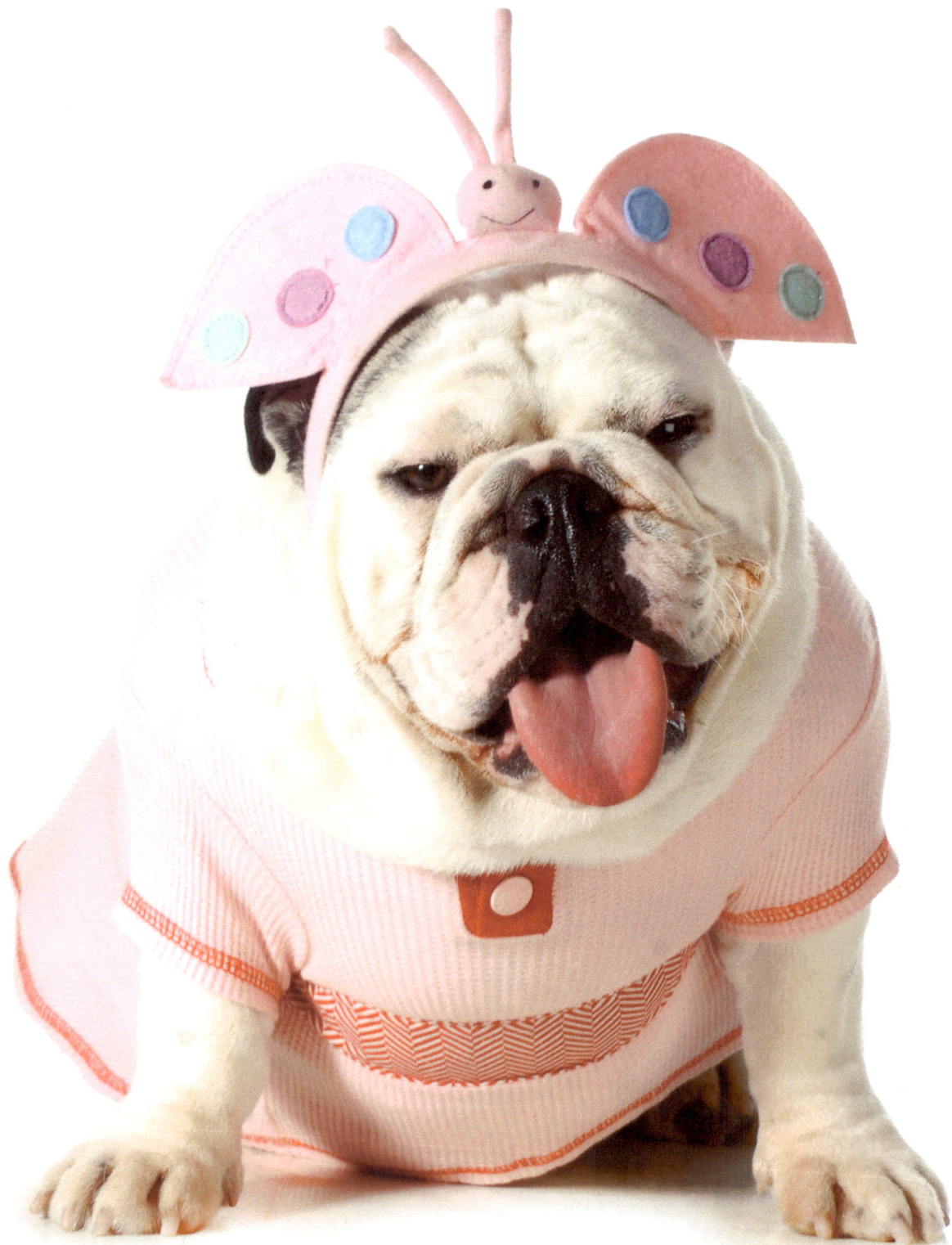

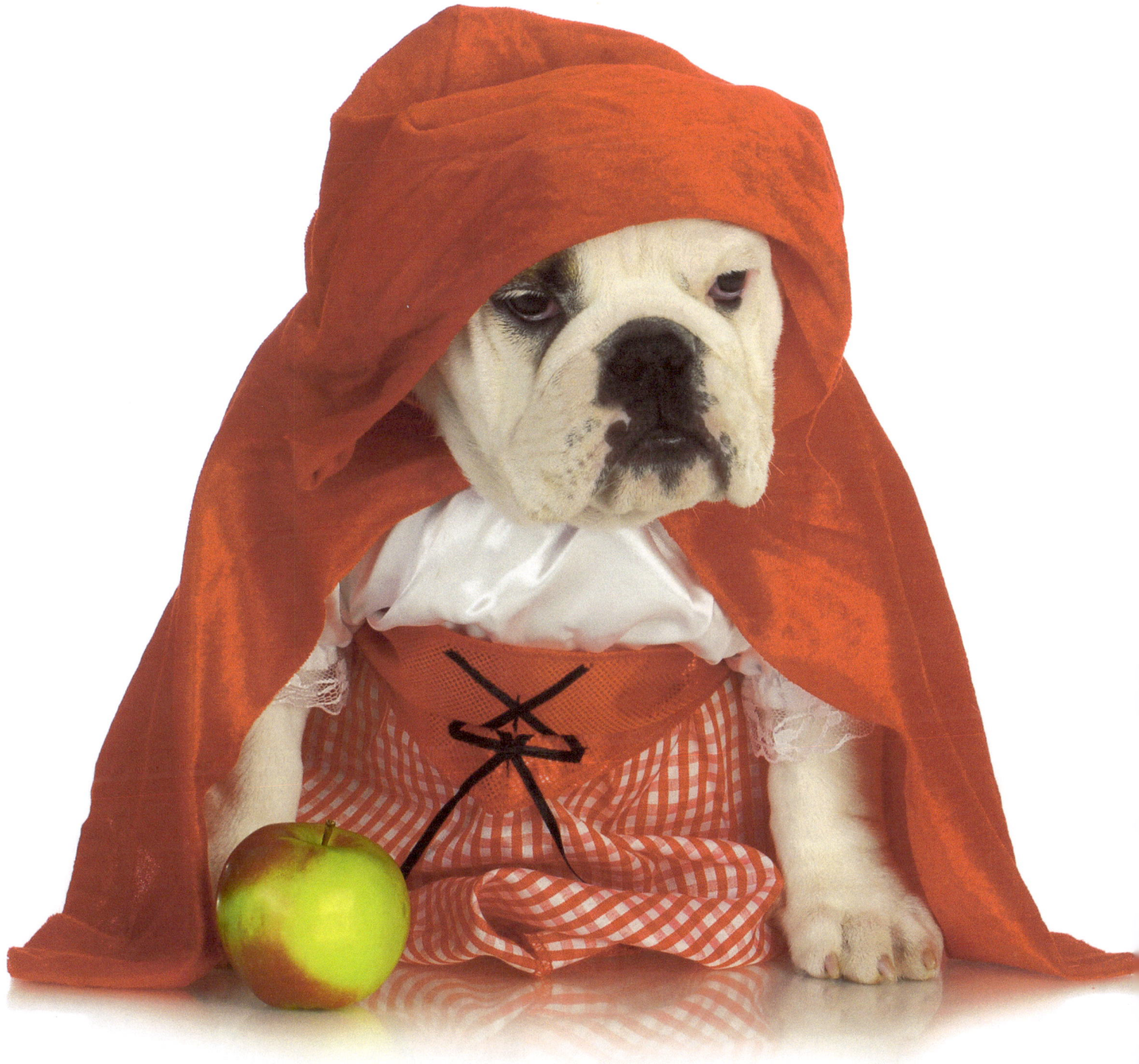

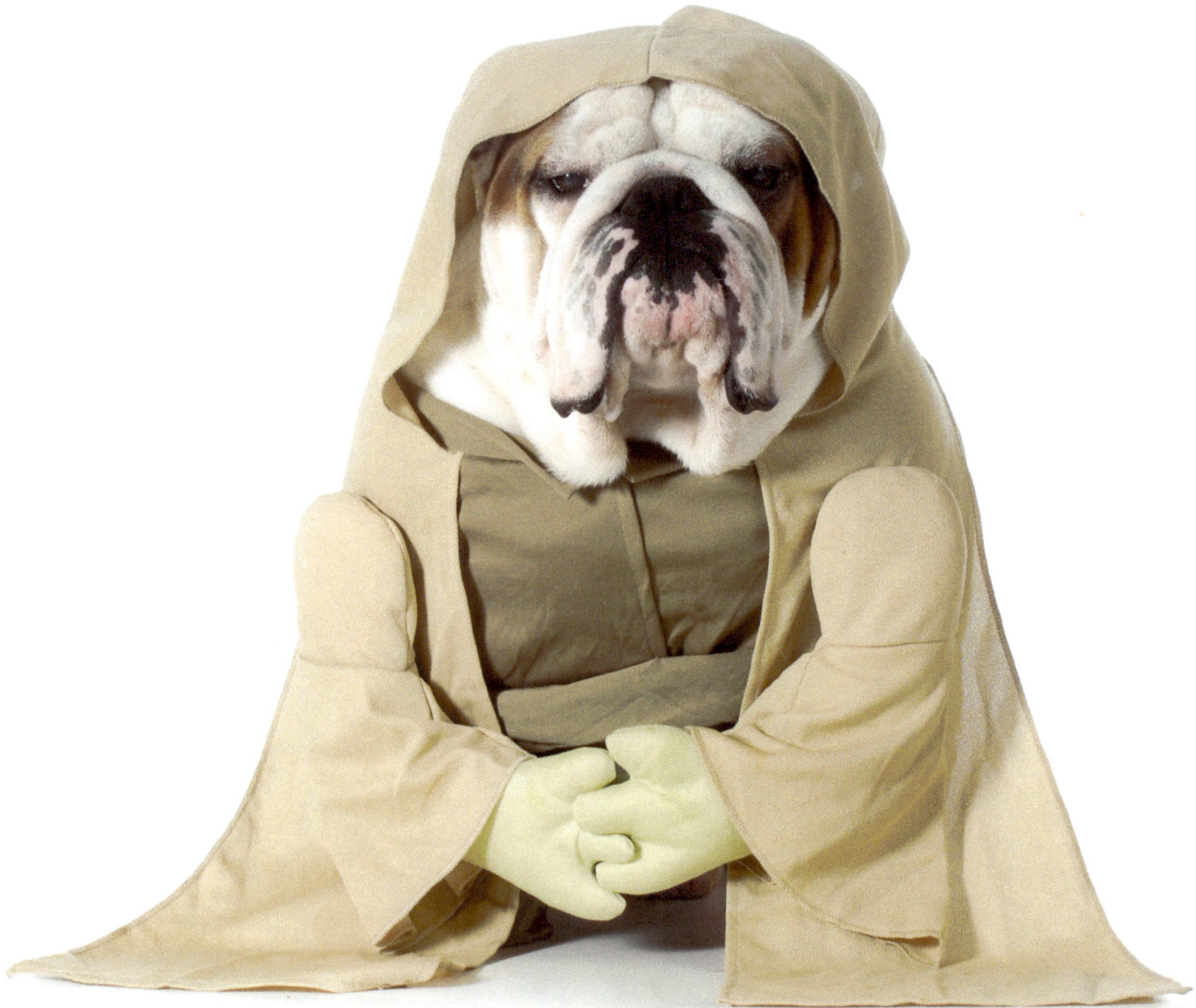

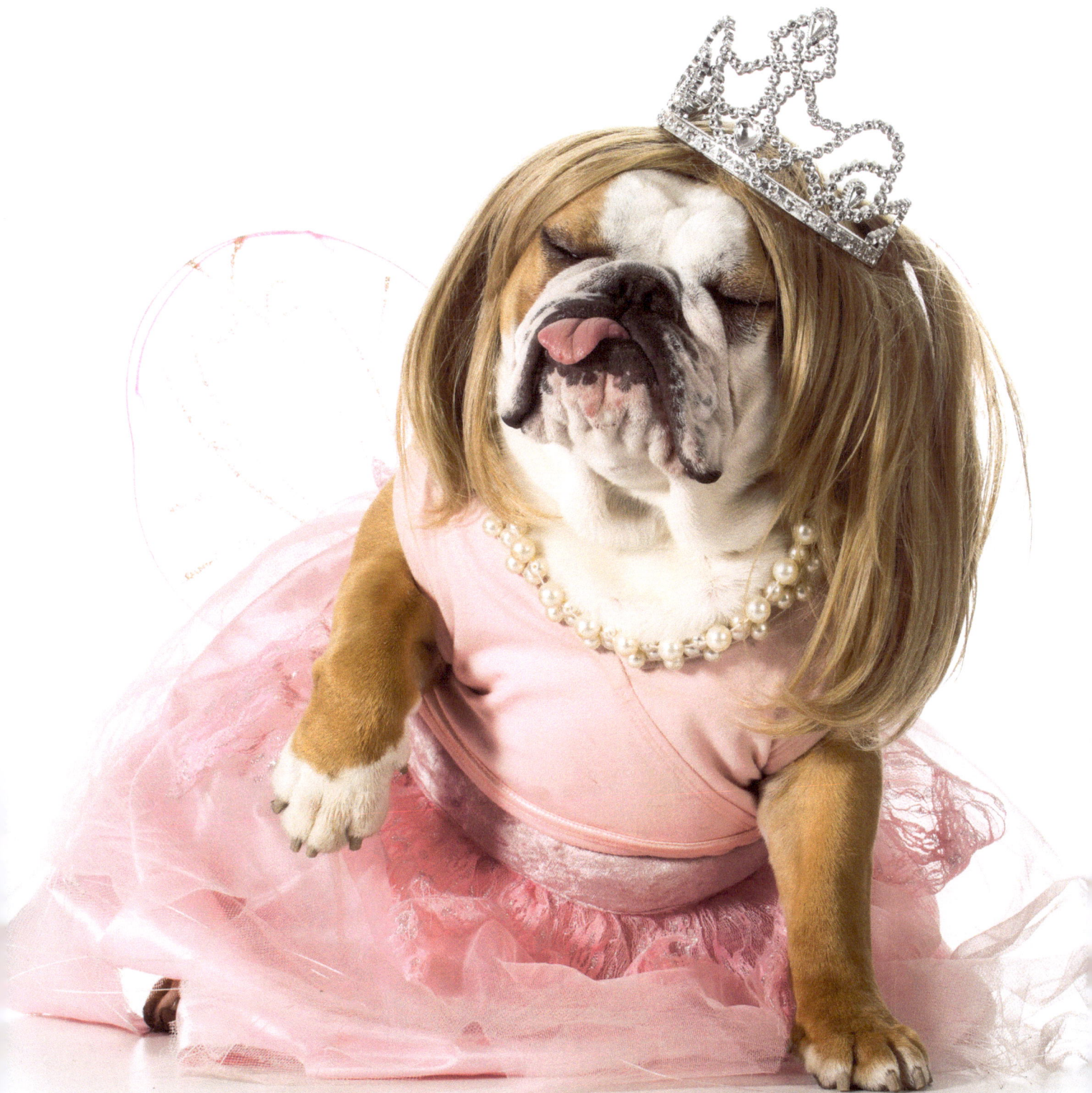

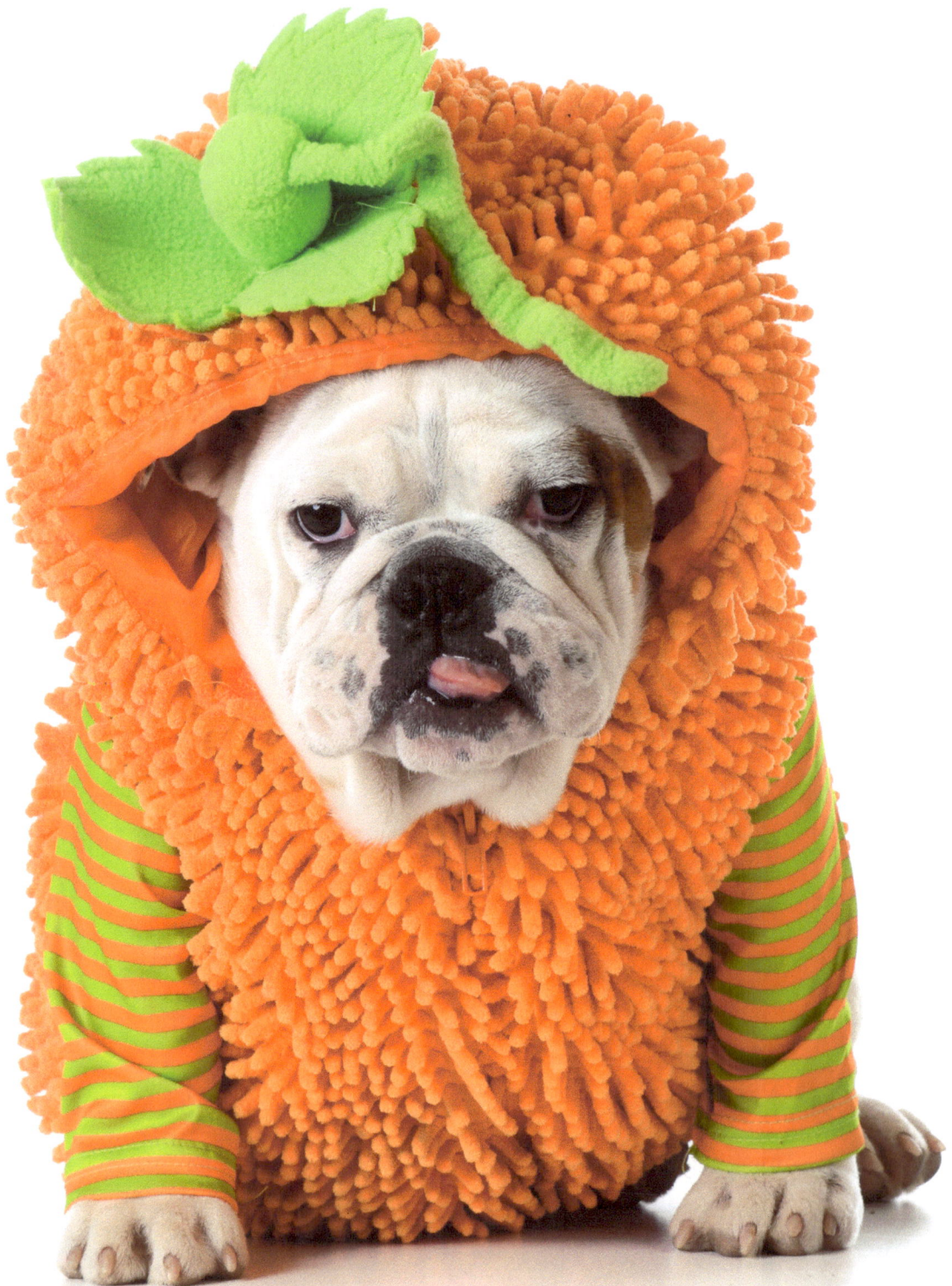

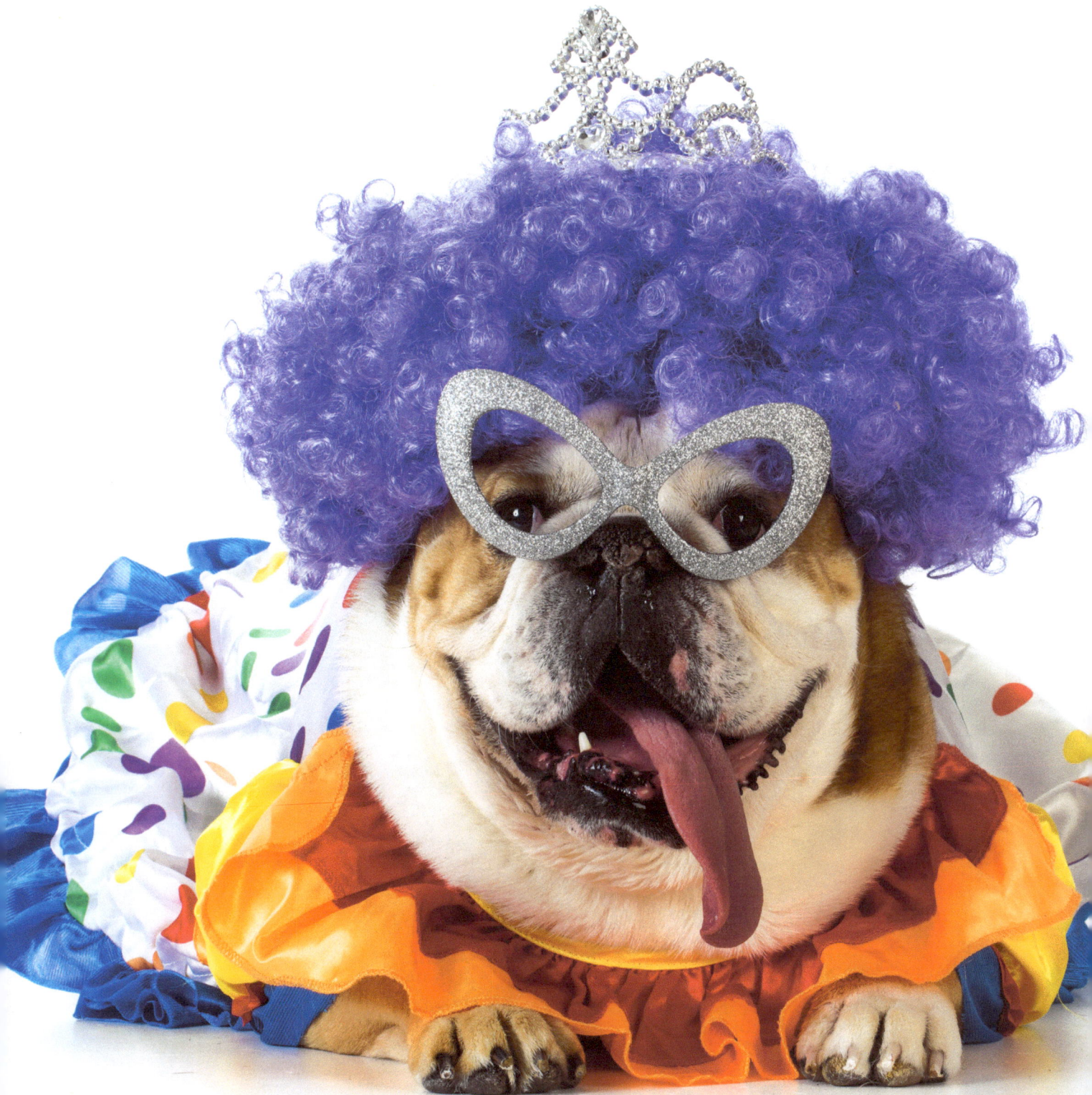

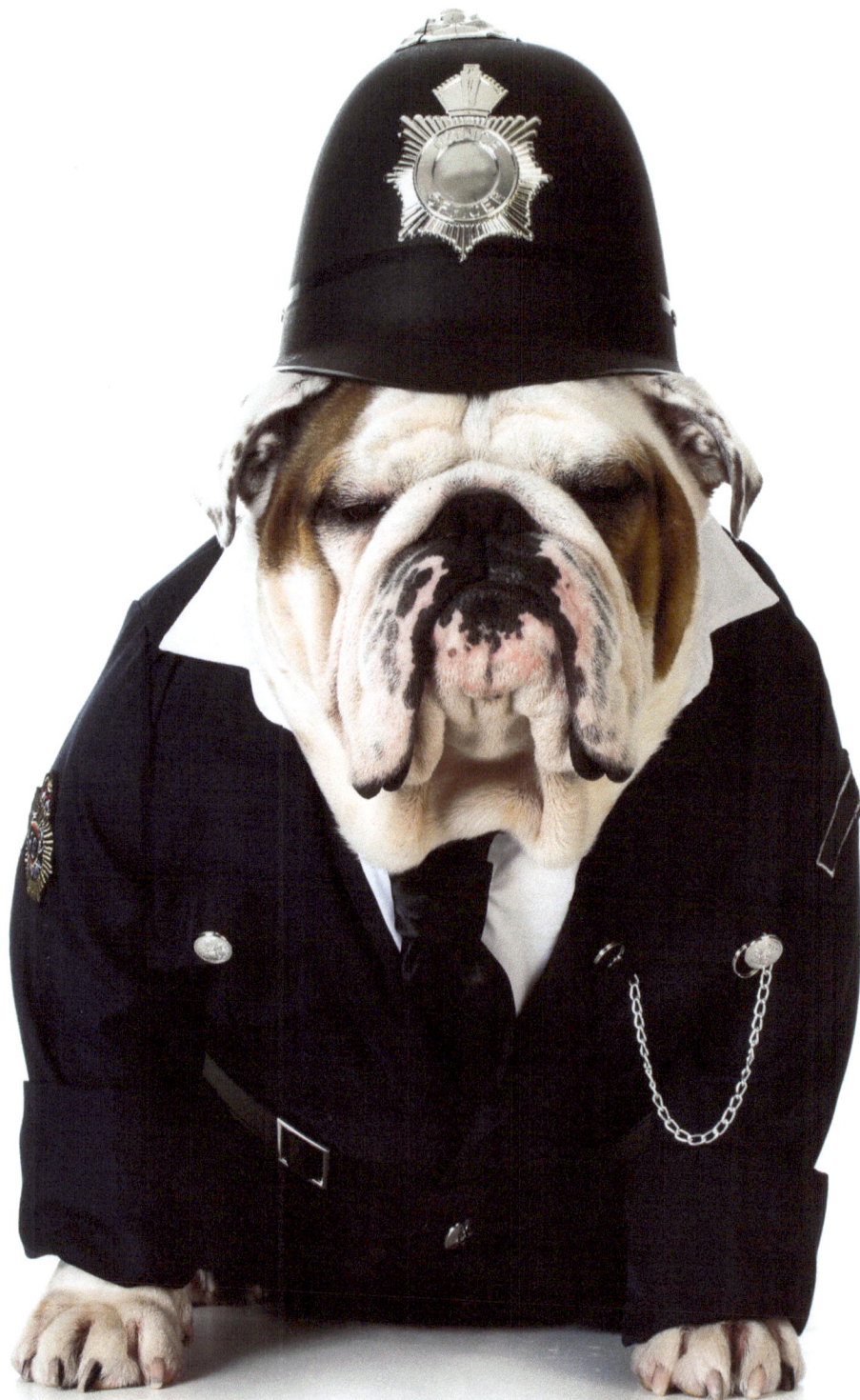

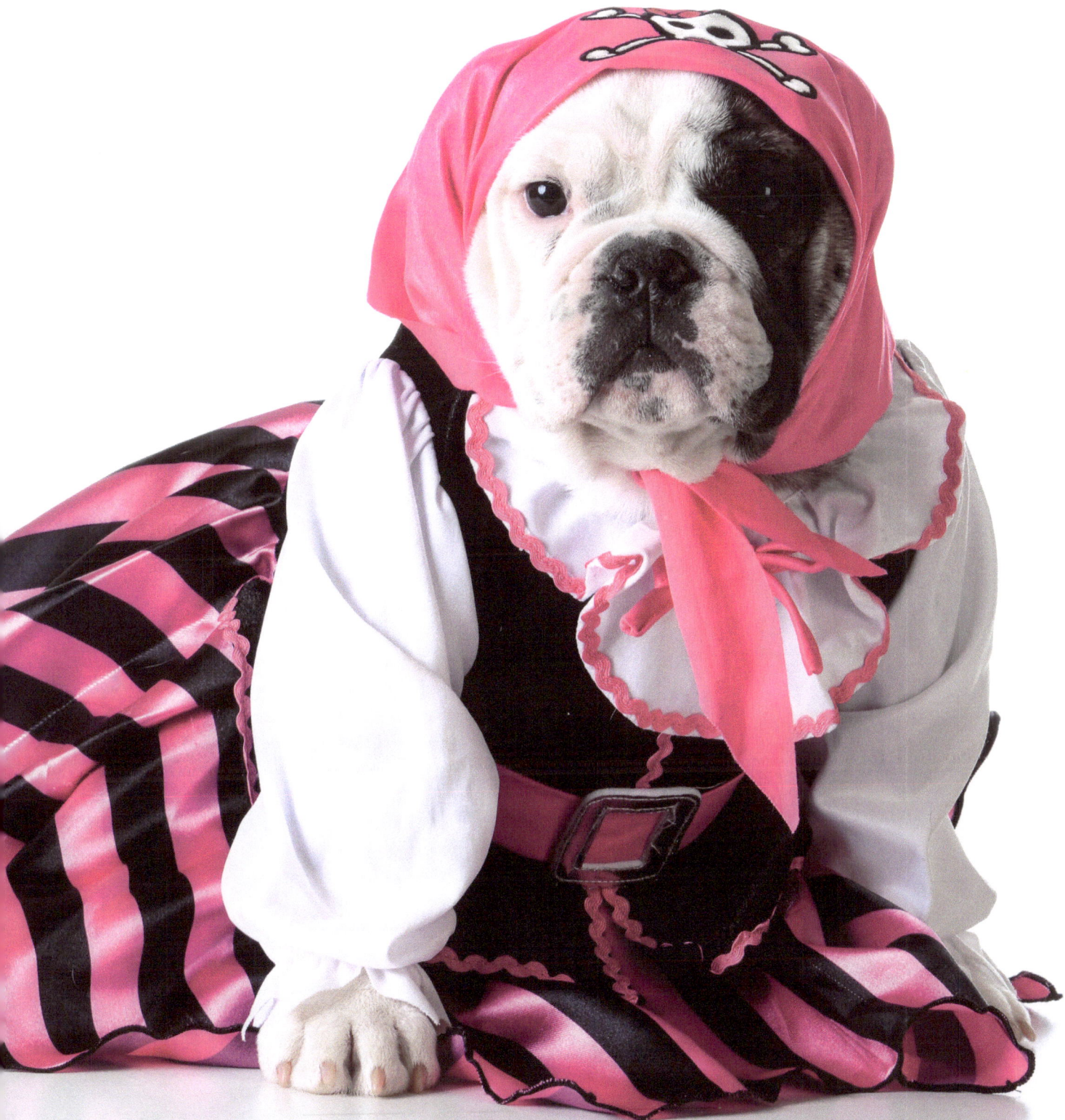

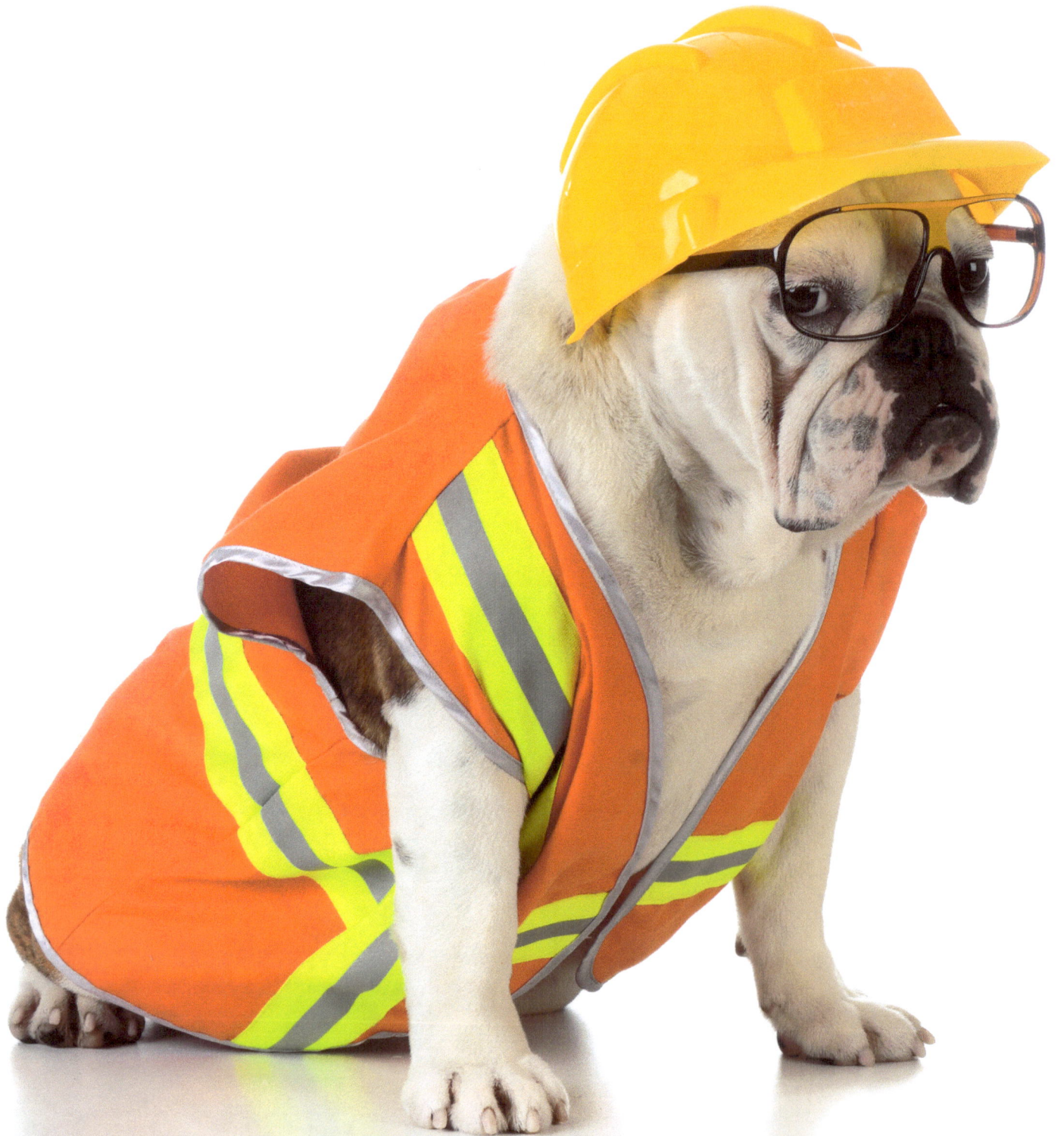

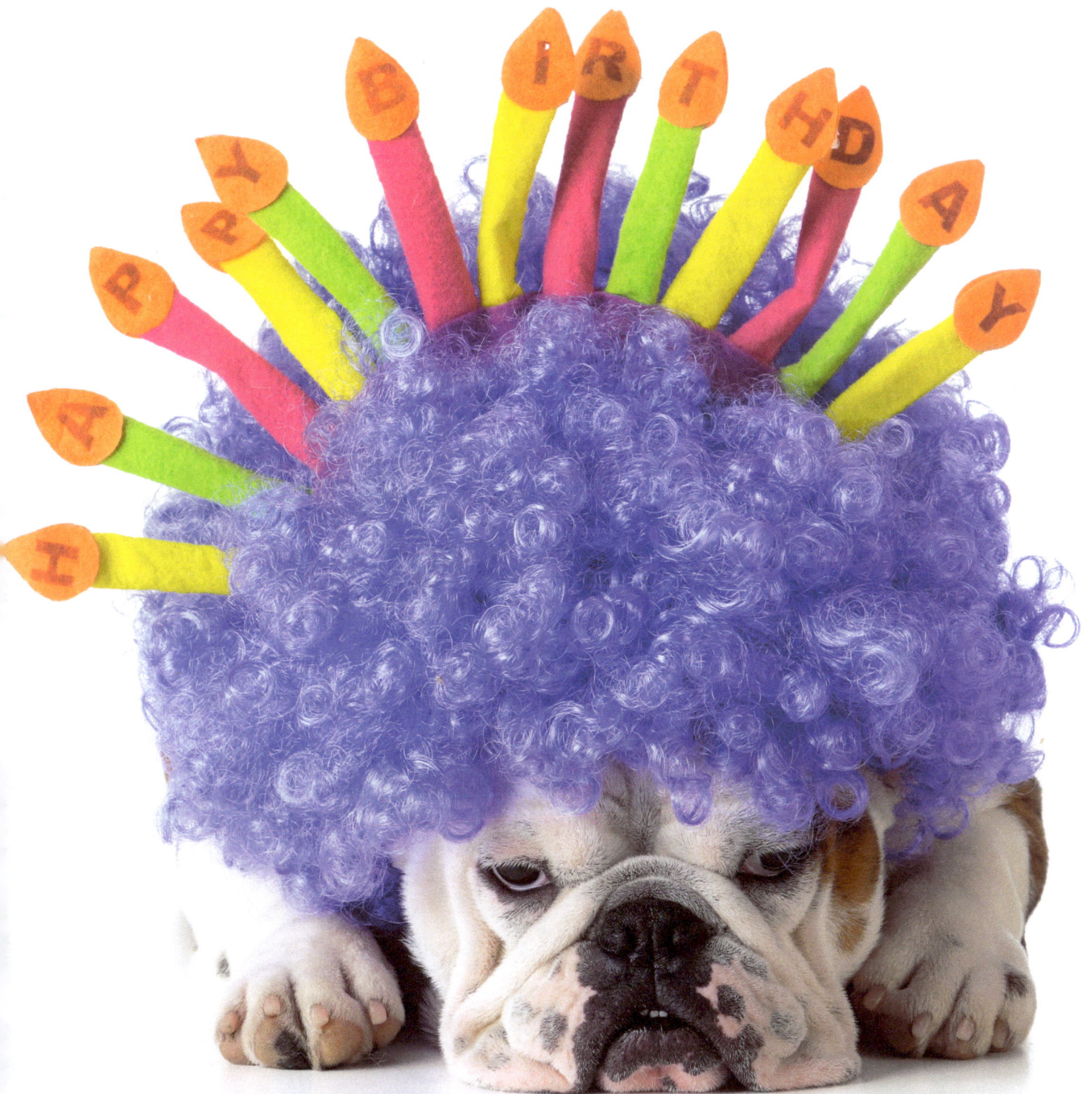

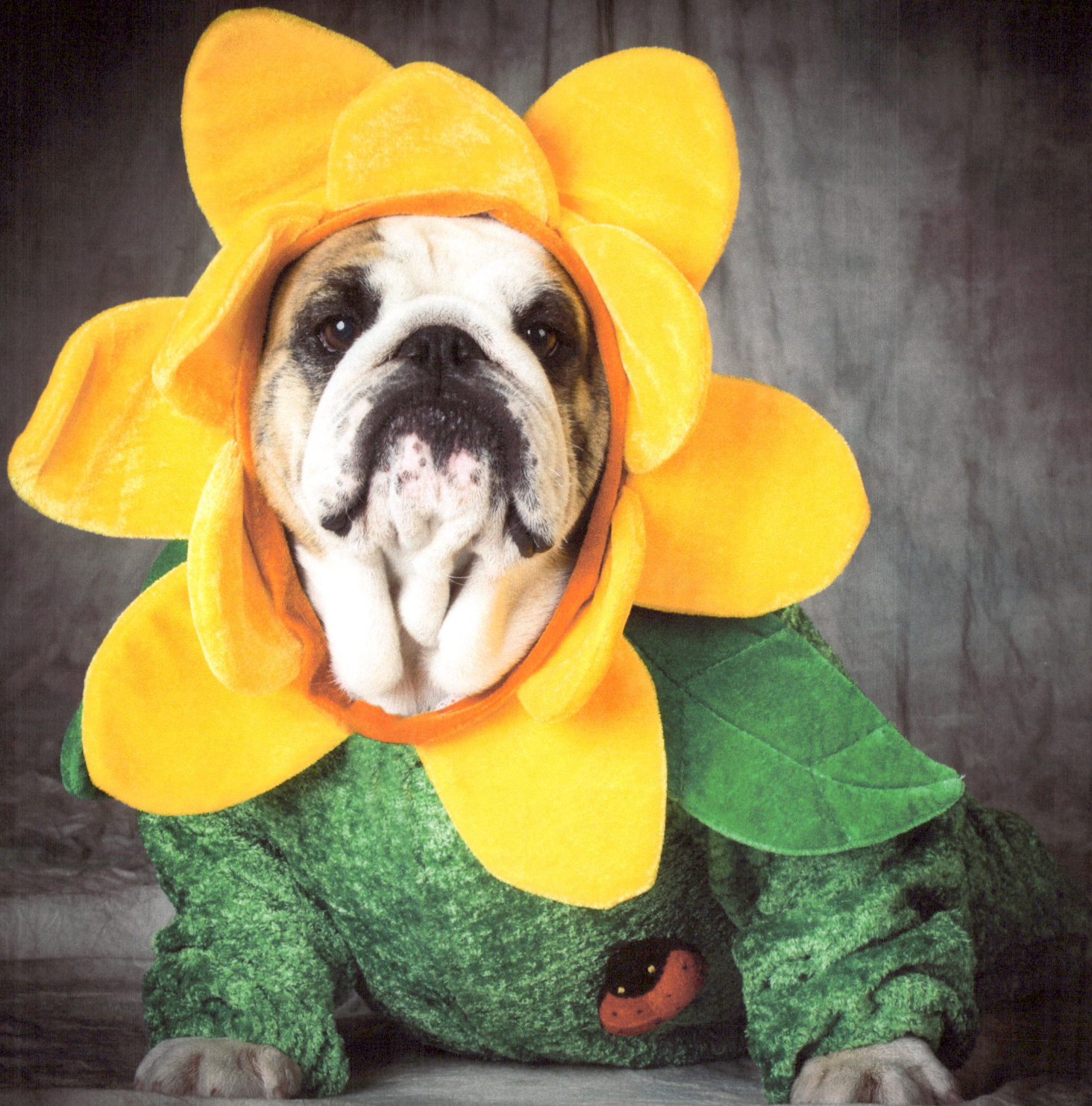

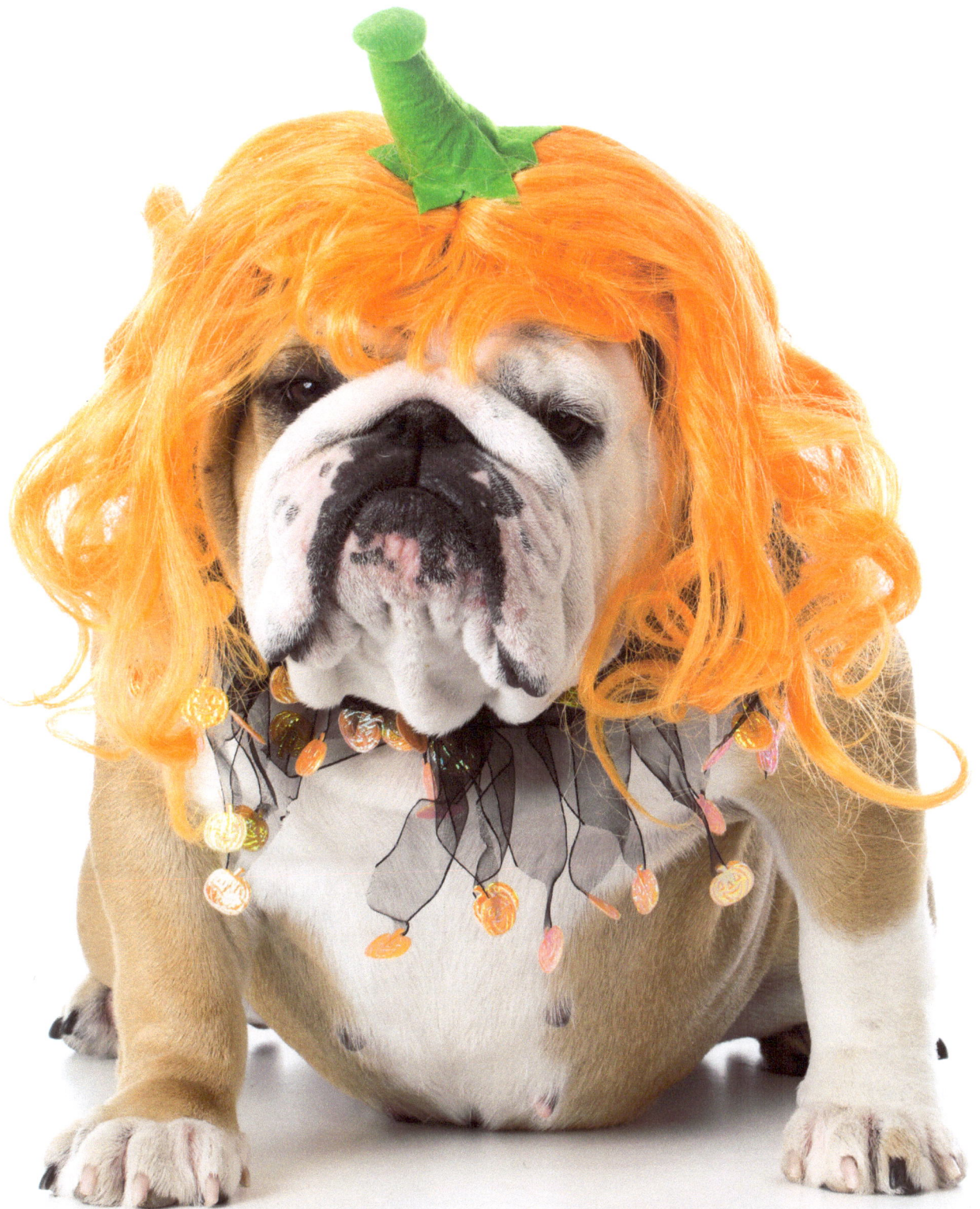

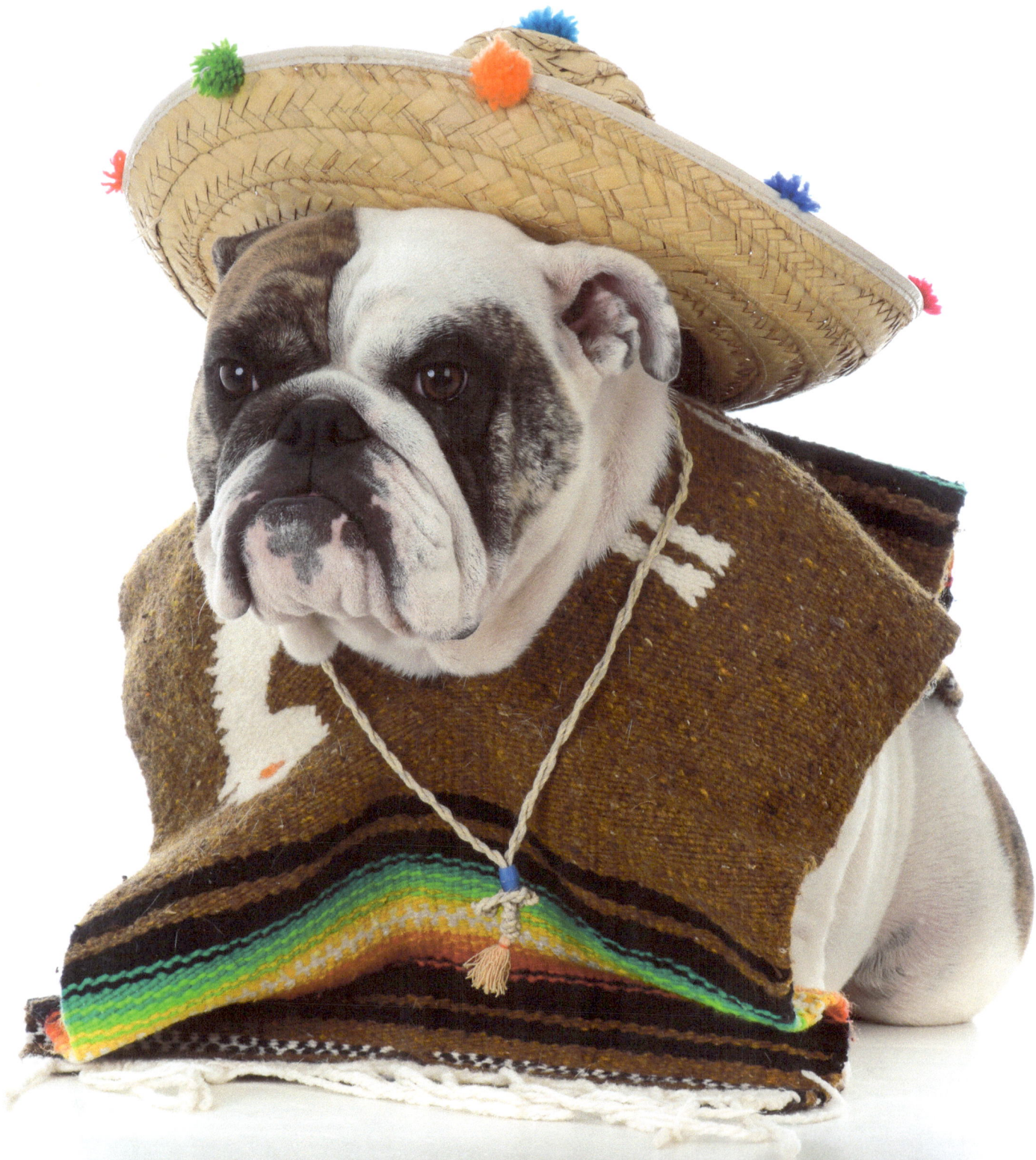

www.ingramcontent.com/pod-product-compliance
Lightning Source LLC
Chambersburg PA
CBHW061143030426

42335CB00002B/78